THE POINTLESS REVOLUTION!

THE ECONOMICS OF DOING WHATEVER YOU WANT

PAUL RANSOM

EVERYTIME PRESS

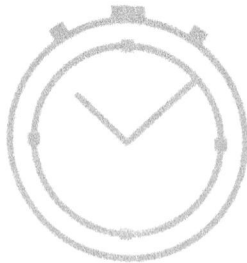

Everytime
Press

The Pointless Revolution! copyright © Paul Ransom
First published September 2019 by Everytime Press

BP#00082

ISBN: 978-1-925536-74-4

Everytime Press
32 Meredith Street
Sefton Park SA 5083
Australia

Email: sales@everytimepress.com
Website: http://www.everytimepress.com
Everytime Press catalogue: https://everytimepress.com/everytime-press-catalogue/

Cover design copyright © Matt Potter
Hourglass image copyright © OpenClipart-Vectors
Watch image copyright © sumoncps
Author photo by Guy Phillips
PHI image by Michelle Cahill

Also available as an eBook:
ISBN: 978-1-925536-75-1

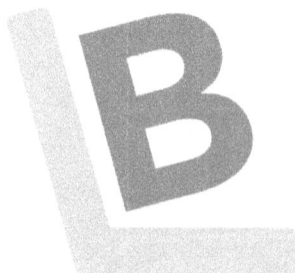

Everytime Press is a member of
the Bequem Publishing collective

https://www.bequempublishing.com/

Although this book is called

THE POINTLESS REVOLUTION!

THE ECONOMICS OF DOING WHATEVER YOU WANT

if you prefer, you can call it

HOW NOT TO BE A SLAVE

THE MEANINGLESS LIFESTYLE GUIDE

EXISTENTIAL ECONOMICS & THE MATHEMATICS OF HAPPINESS

'MEANING' IS A PRISON:
SLAVE NARRATIVES, SYSTEM BLAMING & THE KEY TO FREEDOM

HAPPINESS IS POINTLESS:
HOW TO LIVE A LIFE OF MEANINGLESS PLEASURE

KICK THE BUCKET LIST: LIFE WITHOUT MUSTS & SHOULDS

WHY NOT TO BOTHER (AND JUST BE)

or even

LIVING LIGHTLY: SHED THE SHOULD, LOSE THE LIST & BE FREE

NB: The author actually wants you to re-imagine & personalise the ideas in this book; so feel free to tear off the cover and re-brand the whole thing.

WARNING!

This book contains counter-intuitive ruminations on the related topics of freedom and happiness. Sacred cows will be (humanely) euthanised, passive assumptions challenged and standard meaning tropes usurped. Dogmatists, economists and spiritualists alike will likely have their safe spaces invaded. There will also be frequent references to death, human frailty and meaning-less voids.

PS: Silver bullets, system blaming excuses and enlightenment pathways not included.

CONTENTS

PREFACE

A point to consider before proceeding:
I embarked on the process this book outlines
without knowing what the outcome would be.
May the revolution deliver for you as it did for me.

I am manifestly unqualified to write this book. I have no formal training in economics, psychology, neuroscience or philosophy. In fact, as I type, it would be fairer to suggest that my real qualification is as a failed artist. Despite decades of effort I have no best seller or cult classic to my name and I am yet to direct my much dreamt about debut feature. I live in abject obscurity. I am small fry. Make that tiny fry.

And yet … I enjoy an abundance of liberty. Indeed, I am one of the richest people I know. For I do not own an alarm clock. Nor a tie. I get up when I like, do cool arty things that I mostly enjoy, go to my favourite café more or less whenever I choose and rarely ever need to endure the rush hour. My total debt is below a thousand and thus far my health has been kind to me – steadily failing eyesight* notwithstanding.

(* Although I was born with a basket of herditary eye problems – myopia, cone dystrophy, colour blindness and others – I was diagnosed as being 'legally blind' in 2017, part way through writing this book.)

True, I don't have a lot of stuff; nor do I have the funds for exotic travel, fancy dinners or guitar pedals. I've been cutting my own hair for more than a decade and I've taught myself to prepare a range of relatively tasty, low cost vego soups and sauces for when things get really tight.

And of course, I could never afford a girlfriend. Let alone the latest iThing.

But the fact is, I love the lightness of living this way. I love that my time is principally my own; and I shake my head and smile when people tell me how assiduously they're working their arse off for the better life they've imagined. For their name in lights or their comfy retirement villa. So they can tick items off their bucket list. Or worst of all, so they can attain a pristine state of enlightenment or vibrate themselves to nirvana.

Whatever else you may glean from this book, I can assure you of one thing only. Namely, that the approach I will outline herein works beautifully for me. And really, all I'm doing is sharing it with you. Because maybe it will work for you as well – and then you too can afford to be free.

After all, isn't that why you're reading this?

PS: A note on language.

I have deliberately chosen to use provocative terminology and to sprinkle a few profanities throughout. (So fuck yeah, to some degree I *am* trying to jolt you.) In addition, I have also employed 'parentheses' quite a bit, if only to dilute the tendency of pedants and semantic purists to take up a deliberately narrow view. Where you see 'quote marks' I invite you to take a broader view and connect with the spirit of what I'm saying, rather than limit yourself to dictionary definition.

INTRODUCTION

It's the existential economy, stupid!
Because getting the life budget
in the black is a matter of time;
and happiness is the heretical bottom line.

The spark for this book came from a throwaway comment. My father and I were talking on the phone and I happened to make reference to an earlier episode in my life, right after the meltdown of my fourteen year marriage.

I had skipped the city and gone to live in the tropics, leaving a safe job, a great house and nearly all my worldly possessions behind.

"Gee, that was a waste of time, wasn't it?" he said casually, as if the truth of his assertion were self-evident.

Generally I allow such things to pass without much more than a grin and a (hipsterish) eye roll but on this occasion I felt moved to challenge. "Really? Why's that?"

His response predictably rested upon assumptions about the primacy of career, the notion that achievement is a merely vocational outcome and, of course, the all-conquering pragmatism of money.

My comeback went something like this: "I dunno Dad, three years walking barefoot on a beautiful palm fringed beach and strolling about in the pristine rainforest, whilst never once needing a house key, a jacket or a pair of sensible shoes doesn't sound so bad to me."

To his eternal credit, Dad got the point and the conversation moved on. But the gist of it remained. A lid had been lifted. A fundamental question accidently asked. What does it mean to waste time; and furthermore, what is the true value of time?

That evening I continued to ponder the underpinning values that fuelled my father's critique; to tease out the often unchallenged beliefs that lead so many of us to choose work over play and to pursue status and success so relentlessly that we are prepared to sacrifice ethics, health and relationships to the gods of power, wealth and acclamation.

Of course, there are explanations aplenty for this. Insights exist in evolution, psychology, neuroscience and in the way our societies are organised. Even New Age salvation junkies and their doomsday prepping cousins in the conspiracy scene have 'reasons' to offer. Indeed, thousands of practical, critical and nominally rational narratives exist to make sense of our almost universal submission to a set of received values that most of us – when we stop to think about them – *don't actually believe.*

Then again, if we're honest, we all sacrifice privately held values to publically approved ones. We do this because we're scared. Of disapproval. Of failure. Of going without. In a world where fame and fortune equal fuckability, where being endlessly busy is a badge of honour, and the Joneses not only have to be kept up with but thoroughly gazumped in the 'must have' stakes, it seems more prudent to play along than to nick off to a rainforest and risk getting your feet dirty.

The standard issue response here is 'I have no choice' but, let's be frank, for the vast majority of us living in the comfortably complacent First World, this is an excuse. More than that, it is an abdication. A way to avoid responsibility. A psychological sleight of hand that lets us blame others – parent, partner, boss, bank, etc – for anything we don't like. If we wake up every morning and find ourselves on a treadmill it is because we have *chosen* the rat race; because we have opted to place a higher value on looking the goods and getting the stuff than we have on living in other ways.

That said, I am prepared to concede that this is a very easy thing to assert. I will also allow for the fact that so much of what passes for 'alternative' is little more than a pose and that most of the self-righteous bullies who bore the rest of us senseless with their endless crusading and knee jerk oppositional stance on everything are in fact propping up the very status quo they claim to be questioning. Because, just like the weary commuter/consumer who feels they have no choice, they too are arguing for their own slavery and blaming others for their ill-fitting chains.

Thus, you will doubtless be glad to learn that this book will *not* seek to convince you that everything you know is a lie. Neither will it look to mandate a pathway to paradise or implore you to give up blue cheese, beating off or watching the footy.

Instead, these pages will offer you a bunch of pretty simple ideas culled from personal experience and propped up by stuff I've co-opted from economics, psychology and politics. (With a dash of armchair Existentialism for added spice.)

All of which brings me back to my dad and his 'waste of time' comment; and in particular the cultural and economic imperatives underwriting it. What Dad really meant was that ducking off to a small town in the hotbox of the tropics interrupted the linear momentum of my sensible city-based career and cost me thousands – and he was dead right about that. It did. Decamping to the Coral Sea was, to some extent, financial and professional suicide. In fact, I have still not recovered the lost ground.

But here's the thing. I no longer care to. Or not so much anyway. The reason is simple. I value something else more highly.

Time.

In other words, the days and nights I have left until … well y'know, that time. Given this, I am, at fifty three, not so keen to waste much more of it. Rather, I now prefer to spend it wisely. (As I'm sure you do yours.)

Whilst this may seem little more than cosy fireside hokey, there is an opportunity waiting for us in the wording. *Spend* it wisely.

Okay, so let's park the 'wisely' part for the moment and turn our attention to the 'spend' bit. How would it be if we placed an economic value on our time? God no! I hear you scream. Keep your commodifying hands off my mortality.

But before you close the cover and send this volume to the 'later' pile, let me assure you that what I am proposing here is not for you to sell your soul to the bank but to have the banker recognise your soul's value; and to do so by co-opting *their* belief system. In other words, I am going to plant a freak flag on Wall Street and run the risk metrics over the most valuable asset any of us have.

Just as we now believe it appropriate to price pollution and to recognise the so-called triple bottom line – fiscal, social, environmental – this book will investigate what might happen if we genuinely priced our time. (And I don't mean just jacking up our hourly rate.) How differently would we invest the ever decreasing supply of this asset if we could rescue it from the cotton wool clutches of what we loosely call 'spirituality' and give it a measurable value?

On one hand this is a relatively simple conceptual adjustment, on the other a double-sided heresy; injecting humanity into the economy and much needed rigour into the intellectual void of spiritual cliché. My expectation here is that both the hippies and the corporates will have their respective feathers ruffled.

Indeed, in this book, I will treat economic rationalists and suburban shamans in the same way; as ideologues wedded to a framework that imposes a narrative on the world. And of course, I too will indulge in a little creative framing; it's just that my frame will seek to strip away the excess baggage of meaning and morality and flesh out a much more straightforward proposal for potential happiness.

Yes, happiness. Not simply the pursuit of fun, thrills and other sugar highs but a longer lasting sense of living the life you would prefer rather than the one you believe you have to. Call it joy or contentment if you wish. Or, if you're the more philosophical type, a life of meaning. Hell, you can even call it enlightenment, if you insist. Point being, this book aims to present a way of thinking about the rest of your life that is devoid of religious waffle, righteous pressure and supernatural agency.

NB: A note on happiness.

Before we go any further, let's clarify what I mean by happiness and why I've elected to use this word instead of terms like wisdom or wellbeing.

Clearly, I am attracted to happiness because its use ruffles people. Happiness, it would appear, has an image problem. It is widely regarded as the idiot cousin of healthy, wealthy and wise – the shallow but good looking friend of love and other noble endeavours. My deliberate employment of the term has, I'm pleased to report, already stirred the sediments amongst the early readers of this book. Looks like happiness isn't a lofty enough goal for them. Their preferences have fallen more into the 'life of meaning' basket. Happiness obviously didn't sound like a sufficiently serious and uplifted objective. Too low brow maybe.

However, aside from using it to poke at your assumptions, my choice of the H word stems from a profound yet astonishingly simple question. Is it the enlightenment or sense of meaning we crave or is it, rather, the feeling states we imagine they will engender? What, for instance, is the pay-off of meaning? What is it that enlightenment delivers? In the end, what is all our striving for? What the fuck do we *actually want*?

Even though this opens up a chicken/egg discussion, not to mention the possibility that we're really just quibbling over language, I pose these questions now because they point at a bedrock issue for many of us, which is not really how rich or clever or groovy we seem to be but how we *actually feel* about ourselves and the life we are currently leading.

Throughout the book I will keep coming back to this. What *is* our reality, as opposed to our various fantasies about how it once was or might one day be? *Fuck it, am I happy doing this or not?* Quite aside from whether you think your life is meaningful, does the pursuit and realisation of that so called meaning bring you a deep seated, ongoing sense of happiness? Is the time you're investing in your wisdom/meaning project netting you the dividend of doing whatever you want?

By using the dreaded H word I am also looking to 'keep it real'. Hang all that nonsense about the soul's journey to ultimate understanding or the virtuous trinkets of self-improvement – let alone the obvious vanities of socially visible status and the righteous stench of apparent purity. In the end, I'm much more concerned with *how it feels*. I mean, *really* feels.

So why, you ask, turn to economics?

It's a good question. After all, economics is a cobbled together, pseudo-science which often lurches into vicious, anti-human reductionism. At the altar of the economy we have disrupted the balance of the ecosphere that sustains us, reduced democracy to an infantile farce and produced a brain dead, plastic coated celebrity culture that insults us all. In addition, economists have an abysmal record of predicting stuff – surely a huge KPI fail for them – not to mention a well-documented tendency to over-rely on 'modelling'.

Yet, when we strip away the hubris, greed, and Machiavellian manipulation so often associated with the world of finance, and we look past the failings of the theorists, we find an amazingly useful conceptual skeleton.

In its marrow, economics is about human behaviour. More particularly it is a way of analysing choice. It is also a way of understanding the aggregation that is society. In a very real way, the economy is a map of our co-existence and, in the case of credit, a measure of our trust in one another. Whatever you think about the state of the world right now – good, bad or apocalyptic – remember, we bought it. Individually and collectively.

Economics also provides a powerful way of thinking about uncertainty. Its focus on assessing risk and reward is more useful and honest than anything on offer in any of the world's much cherished spiritual traditions.

Then there is the question of value. What do we actually *mean* by that?

- How and why do we value some things more than other things?
- What are we prepared to trade-off in order to attain this apparently valuable stuff?
- Are there quantifiable ways of measuring and comparing different kinds of value that can help us to make smarter decisions about an uncertain future?

To me, these are incredibly useful tools for thinking about life. Partly, they are wasted on something as monochromatic as money. Maybe we should raid the economists' toolkit and use their intellectual infrastructure to talk about the big stuff. What do we *really* value? How can we reform our personal 'economies' to create what the boffins might call optimal utility? In short, can we use the economic mindset to help us live happier, more deeply rewarding lives?

Absolutely yes we can. And in this book I will endeavour to explain how. Hence the subtitle, *The Economics Of Doing Whatever You Want.*

The simple (but not so silly) suggestion contained in these pages will be that if we include time remaining as a line item in our overall 'life budget' we will reckon the competing values in our lives very differently and this, in turn, may well lead us to a radical re-structure. Hell, we might even start doing what we truly enjoy.

Thus, my father was both right and wrong. Time can indeed be wasted but if quitting your safe job and moving to a beach house in the tropics brings more joy to you than a promotion, a new car or the approval of your peers then it may well be that your most economical choice would be to shrug off those corporate shoulder pads, go without the next iFetish and leave your so-called friends to their superannuated servitude.

Gee, wouldn't that be nice?

1.

HOURGLASS ECONOMICS

or

Understanding the true value of your time

You know damn well that a shiny new car or luxury apartment won't fulfil you. That being top dog won't bring you the love you want. That fame is a vanity – a tacky star on a footpath somewhere – and that power comes hand in glove with the fear of losing it. So why are you spending your time chasing it?

In this chapter I identify the central denial at work in human cultures, examine the way in which it plays out in our personal lives and argue that by regarding time as our most valuable life asset and adopting the conceptual toolkit of economics, we can create a practical framework for happiness.

T here are clues aplenty in everyday language about the fundamental value of time. Mostly we throw such comments away. They are clichés. We say them and soon forget what they are telling us.

- Spending time.
- Time is money.
- Quality time.
- Free time.
- My time is valuable.
- That's an hour I won't get back.

Yet at some point in our lives most of us will have our time monetised in the form of hourly rates, per diems, annual salaries, time in lieu, overtime, etc. The idea of time being a finite resource that should be paid for by those who wish us to use it up for their benefit – typically employers – is both universally accepted and utterly banal.

So why do most of us routinely waste it? Why do we offer up our best years to perform tasks we'd rather not for arseholes we don't really like? Why does the professional so often take precedence over the personal? What drives us to keep postponing the life we would rather lead in order to uphold a Faustian pact with money, status and objects?

The reasons for this include personal, social, ethical, cultural and hardcore financial factors – and although each of us negotiates these tugs on our time differently, there exists an almost universal tendency for us to sacrifice the present to an imagined future.

How often have you heard the following kinds of narrative offered up as reasons – or indeed excuses?

- I'll work hard now and live it up later.
- If I make the money now I'll be able to provide a better future for my family.
- Just a couple more years and I'll …
- Once I pay off the house, I'll …
- Oh c'mon, honey, I'm doing this for us.

My intention here is not to blithely dismiss the notion of working and persevering – or indeed to minimise the very real and immediate pressure that lack of adequate finance can place upon people – but rather to underline our often unconscious costing of time and our frequently poor grasp of risk assessment.

These habits begin when we first come to understand that we will one day die – or when we discover that there is a real difference between the thing we call work and the thing we call play. Even as children we treasure our weekend and school holiday time. Then, as we move into adulthood and the decades tick by, we begin to notice the undeniable arrow of time. We see it and feel it in our bodies. We watch it speeding by as our parents decline and our kids grow. For most of us there comes a day when we can no longer hold back the idea that time spent has begun to outweigh time remaining.

Once again, universal and banal – except that as a species we have wrapped this realisation in layers of denial. We know we're doomed but we act like we have forever. We understand that everything is in a state of flux, yet we dedicate ourselves to the delusion of permanence. Pretty well every spiritual and religious tradition offers its adherents a palliative for their mortality – afterlives, reincarnations, etc – and today science is increasingly holding out hope that we will one day be able to dodge time's deadly bullet with pills, cryogenic suspension and other such fountains of eternal youth. And then there's our penchant for grand monuments to ourselves – pyramids, palaces and pillars of stone – or the vain allure of immortalising ourselves on film, in song or within the retro-fitted realm we call history. As if these follies will somehow make us less dead. As if eternal life was actually a *good* thing.

Therefore, to say that we have a fear-based culture is, in my view, a crashing understatement. Whilst fear certainly serves an evolutionary purpose and can operate as a useful psychological call to action, it is also the engine of denial – and in the case of our death, our dread powers what I like to call the 'central denial'.

You may well argue that this is a necessary existential sidestep. I mean, if the fact of your death was constantly front row centre in your thoughts you might find yourself disinclined to pursue grand objectives; never mind getting up on bitterly cold mornings to do some spirit crushing job for nowhere near enough money. Indeed, you might even lapse into the kind of fatalistic, 'fuck it all' mentality that lends itself to the casual excusing of injustice and the ill-treatment of others. Clearly, a level of judicious forgetting is both personally and socially beneficial.

NB:

I will outline a more positive and liberating compromise with mortality in Chapter 5.

However, our culture and our economy have elevated this denial to the point of hubris. From the asinine, bourgeois arrogance of the New Age to the virgin-packed heaven of suicide bombers, we have concocted an array of death-defying narratives that have unleashed all manner of cruelty, greed and needless sorrow on the world. How many people have we put to the sword in the name of our favourite brand of eternity? How many cool millions have been banked by those selling this paradise or that paradigm to suckers and seekers everywhere?

Conspiracy nerds would say that 'the system' requires both the denial and the divide and conquer social architecture that most often accompanies it in order to keep us focused on buying false hope and competing with one another for trinkets and status. To an extent I agree. Even though the competitive instinct and its cohorts – tribalism, territoriality and acquisitiveness – are deeply rooted in our evolution, it is apparent that there *are* those who cynically exploit these proclivities for power and profit.

Yet regardless of where we sit on the conspiracy spectrum, the absent presence here is our finite and dwindling supply of time. Traditionally, most of us have regarded this asset in stubbornly vague terms. Whether we tell ourselves that we're an immortal spirit manifesting in human form or that we're simply a vessel for a cabal of selfish genes, we generally baulk at the idea of bringing any serious rigour to the weighing up of time. In my view, this is part of what allows us to continue in denial – and thus to keep on working and striving for stuff we already know won't make us happy.

You know damn well that a shiny new car or luxury apartment won't fulfil you. That being top dog won't bring you the love you want. That fame is a vanity – a tacky star on a footpath somewhere – and that power comes hand in glove with the fear of losing it. So why are you spending your time chasing it?

Here in the West at least, pundits typically insult our intelligence with superficial spirituality and Oprahfied pop-shrinkery whenever we address this question. They say stuff like *everything happens for a reason* or they urge us to align ourselves with our divine higher purpose. They may even try to inspire us with idiotic memes on Facebook. All of these are simply the central denial re-packaged – and none of them help us to get to grips with the temporal bottom line.

Indeed, all the while we relegate/elevate our impermanence to the fuzzy firmament of metaphysics we can effectively ignore the blunt truth of it and, by extension, fail to take proper account of our limited time – and in the shadow of this failure, toil pointlessly to achieve meaningless goals.

So here's another question for you. Suppose we took a much cherished article of spiritual orthodoxy and turned it on its head? What if our habitual pursuit of worldly goods and peer approval is not fuelled by the imperial triumph of a supposedly masculine, linear, materialist view of the world but rather by our apparently enlightened refusal to deal honestly with the fact of death? Imagine how different things might be if we

The Central Denial

Our universal proclivity to deny that we are animals and, hence, to pretend that we do not die. By denying our mortality we fundamentally divorce ourselves from 'nature' – which we then cast as an externality. Thus, by regarding death as our enemy we pathologise our essential human condition; and this often maps out in the punishment (sinner/victim) narratives of religion, the moralising control mantras of karma and custom, and the 'immortality' delusions of fame and legacy. In addition, it underwrites and legitimises all standard 'life meaning' tropes and the reductionist, pass/fail criteria they so routinely apply.

brought the central denial down from the clouds and examined it without the drama of moral meaning or the associated fantasy of self-importance. If you could look in the mirror and see yourself as an animal, a thing of nature, rather than a light-filled being floating above or beyond it, what would that imply about the rest of your life?

Like me, many of you are probably already asking yourself what you really want from your remaining years. What really matters to you? What would you like more of? Less of? These are entirely valid questions. The very ones that prompted this book.

Thus, in the shadow of fifty, I turned my full attention to them, believing they required an honest examination, as opposed to something wrapped in wishful thinking and spiritual egomania – and this is where Hourglass Economics sprang from.

Although briefly tempted by the current middle class fashion for lazily co-opting First Nation cosmologies and cherry picking physics for post-Newtonian notions of time and space, I asked myself whether these modalities (and others like them) were the best tools for ascertaining what I truly, deeply valued and, furthermore, what might offer me a genuinely better chance of experiencing more happiness and less misery. More freedom and fewer obligations. Less debt and a diminished desire for – and addiction to – approval and objects.

But before I could answer I needed to work out what all this musing was about. It wasn't about ethics or politics and it most certainly had nothing to do with god, destiny or career. No, it was a question about value. In other words, what was more valuable to me and what did the idea of value rest upon?

Although we are all versed in the arithmetic of value as measured in money, we don't usually employ it to think about things in our personal lives. But suppose we did?

Now, before you shriek in horror, I'm not some villainous investment banking type urging you to reduce everything to dollars, cents and objective utility function. Nor am I suggesting that things like fulfilling relationships and recreational basket weaving are worthless. In fact, in my view these things are much more valuable than an annual bonus or tick box travel opportunity.

Nonetheless, there is something incredibly powerful about the way that economists engage with their topic. Not so much their particular ideology (Keynesian, monetarist, neo-classical and so on) but the very focus of their analysis. They seek to understand the ascribing of value. They try to figure out how best to account for flux and uncertainty and how these can affect perceived value. And even though economics often tries to impose pristine theoretical abstraction onto an irrational world, it does so knowing that it is seeking to imperfectly describe and predict an incredibly complex ecosystem of individual human choices and the transactions they drive. In a way, it is a kind of psychological mathematics – a 'beautiful set of numbers' that opens a window on the vast web of human social exchange. For all of its real world failings and distasteful tendency to reduce people to numbers, economics poses profound questions and endeavours to answer them in very useful, practical terms.

Economics also dares to deal directly with complexity. To weigh up and sift out competing forces. To factor in imperfect, irrational judgement. To allow for the unpredictable. Smart economists even make room in their theorising for what they call radical uncertainty; namely, unforeseeable developments like disruptive technologies and status quo shattering events in society and politics. It performs this juggling act in order to arrive at best case outcomes – or maximum utility. Not perfection, but simply the best available result.

Put very crudely, economics is an exercise in risk assessment and cost/benefit analysis designed to work out which of the many options out there seems most likely to be the best way forward. (Or should I say, going forward?)

Though we might decry the wolves of Wall Street we should be wary of allowing our righteous outrage to blind us to the gems they carry in the pockets of their expensively tailored suits. Even if you remain convinced that the Rothschilds secretly own everything, or that the Bilderberg Group dictates government policy on a global scale, the economist's philosophical toolbox may yet come to your existential rescue.

So, to return the topic of the rest of your life and how best to live it: how might you use an economist's frame to evaluate the competing pressures on your time?

Here's where we get back to the notion of value – and more particularly, to determining the relative values of the contesting and sometimes diametrically opposing options we have before us. This daily multiple choice test typically includes things like health, work, ambition, fun, ethical considerations, the approval of those we love, the importance of family and relationships, and yes, even the availability of finance. We are continually weighing these things up against each other, prioritising one over the other and then promptly re-ordering these priorities as new circumstances arise or yet another blinding epiphany drops down from the sky.

This process can seem endless and confusing. So much so that many of us would, if pressed, readily confess that one of the most difficult questions to answer with any kind of authority is: *what do we really want in life?* Even if the flipside question – what do we *not* want? – is an easier ask, we're still left fumbling with a squillion options, obligations and

---

The economy is us

The way that we commonly speak of and refer to the so-called 'economy' is analogous to the way we speak of 'nature' – namely, as an externality. However, it seems to me that, like money itself, the economy is a social technology. In other words, economy springs from human interaction; from the individual's pursuit of their own needs and wants and the trades they make with others in the process of that pursuit. Thus, rather than regarding the economy as being imposed on us by elites, I consider it a numerical/statistical read out of the aggregate trust* we have in each other and, by extension, of the things we think of as being utile and/or worth paying for. The economy is a live-time barometer of our social health and we all contribute to the read out. Sure, economic inequality and injustice is rife, and the worship of wealth has distorted our culture, our polity and the biosphere, but that too is something we have chosen, or at the very least, allowed. Whatever you think of the present economic order – remember, *we bought it.*

* Re: trust – the Latin root *credo* (meaning *believe*) is where our term credit comes from. To extend credit is literally to affirm belief, To trust.

15

organisational hurdles. After all, knowing what you want (or don't) and going about getting (or avoiding) it are two (possibly four) quite different things. All of this, however, is reckoning without the elephant.

(Insert massive, slow moving pachyderm capable of trampling everything underfoot.)

Welcome back to time. Tick, tick, tick. Yes folks, that's our lives counting down – and were it not for the pervasive power of the central denial we could all begin to accept with equanimity that the defining fact of our living is our dying. Life derives its beautiful urgency and precious quality from the fact that it will certainly end. Indeed, the very notion of life is meaningless without death and the fantasy of eternal life is fundamentally oxymoronic.

You can soften the edges of this if you like by positing any number of afterlives, higher planes or transubstantiated incarnations but I challenge you to honestly refute the fact of your impending physical death. In the realm of the self-identifying conscious experience in which we find ourselves we will all cease to be. The ego, the episode we call I, will end.

So, even if embracing your *complete* demise is a step too far, it is surely no great leap of imagination to suggest that by far the most valuable, least renewable and increasingly rare asset we each have at our disposal is time remaining.

When we take this fact and wrench it from the grasp of gurus and give it a clear, unambiguous numerical value – as if it were a kind of temporal slush fund – we can truly begin to think clearly about what to do with the rest of our lives.

For what it's worth, I have lately done this and the upshot has been literally life altering. Not a silver bullet or a panacea for everything but a tool for focused reflection that asks direct questions and allows no room for denial. Sure, it also requires brutal honesty to be truly effective – but why the fuck would you lie to yourself? I mean, you wanna be happy, right?

Ah yes – happy. As opposed to wise, admired or perfect. Let alone wealthy, well-dressed and thoroughly entertained.

Unlike the world's great religions and their crystal wielding alternatives, the 'economics of happiness' requires no ideological allegiance or enlightened moral vantage point. You can eat what you like, make love to anyone who wants you to, run marathons or lock yourself into your favourite VR metaverse all weekend. And all according to a formula where *you* plug in the numbers.

But here's the other thing. Unlike those seminars you attended or self-help books you diligently ploughed through, this approach does not promise that happiness will be a unitary unbroken field of permanent uplift and Zen-like calm. The economic modality – with time as its gold standard – views happiness in terms of utility. As the probability of a best potential outcome given a number of inputs. This brand of happiness inevitably contains measures of sadness, frustration and so on – just like real life.

It's prudent here to acknowledge the validity of the standard meme – that happiness is not a destination – an achievement – but an attitude. A way of seeing and being. I am not for one moment suggesting that quantifying the value of your remaining years will automatically deliver happiness but rather that, by doing so, you can begin to run a thorough risk analysis of those years to help you get a genuinely useful perspective on yourself and the things you value.

It has been my experience that this mode of reflection has, in effect, significantly increased my potential for happiness by enabling me to work out where I'm going to focus my best efforts and what kind of people I'd like to spend time with over the following decades – and what and who I'm going to kick to the kerb.

THE TEMPORAL EPHEMERAL ASSET CLASS

So why time? Why not something culled from ethics? I mean, we are talking *value* here, after all.

The answer, as you may have guessed, relates to our mortality, or rather to the dread that surrounds it. Whereas spiritual contemplation allows us to wriggle off the death hook and moral philosophy is invariably couched in subjective and socially received terms, the raw fact of time is both external to our wishes and entirely blind and predictable in its application. It does not play favourites. Does not judge. Will not reward us for effort, talent or beauty. It will act upon the sage as surely as it will upon the fool.

The New Agers and armchair physicists amongst you will surely now remind me about everything from Mayan cycles to Special Relativity as a way of diluting assumptions about objective linear time. However, without pre-emptively dismissing these things I think it's fair to say that all of us *experience* time as a directional progress of 'moments' – as an ongoing analogue process of constant change.

Your reading of this sentence is surely proof enough. Indeed, for you to have *any* experience whatsoever means that you live in linear time. What's more, the very notion of *you* is only possible in a universe where time passes in a predictable, directional fashion and where pattern recognition is possible. Or, to put it in hippy speak, to be incarnated is to manifest in time.

By accepting this in its truest, deepest sense we can begin to see that time is the spine of who we are and everything we will ever think, want and do. We are nothing without it – and when it runs out we will be nothing once more.

This is why time is the ultimate unit of value – and why it is the best candidate for underwriting the relative value of everything else.

Doubtless some of you will be going, *yeah, so what, this is obvious* and I would concur. Much of this has a ho-hum motherhood feel about it. Yet perhaps there is also a 'hidden in plain view' quality to it. So immediate and apparent that we habitually overlook it. How else to explain the plethora of fanciful, denialist stories we tell ourselves about anthropomorphised deities and externally authorised life meanings? If we honestly accepted the primacy of time – and thus, our own mortality – why would we need the fantasy of forever?

Although our attachment to notions of meaning, purpose and self-importance clearly play into this – as does our hardwired survival instinct – I believe that most of us have the intellectual capacity and intestinal fortitude to take the banality of death and use it to create a better life for ourselves.

The sheer impersonal coldness of time – the fact that it does not depend upon our moral fibre, bank balance or ideological disposition for its power – affords us the very external, independent yardstick we look for in gods, destiny narratives and honour culture. Something beyond our own ego. An outside perspective. Our place in the scheme of things.

Lacking both form and substance, it has a dynamic, mathematical and, dare I say, mystical quality that gives it an egalitarian universality that perfectly qualifies it as the reserve currency of existential account. So, how are you going to spend it?

THESE ARE THE DAYS OF OUR LIVES

Let's play a little game. Picture an hourglass. Sands of time and all that. (Days of our lives, if you will.) Flip it over and, hey presto, the grains start dropping.

At the start of the game you don't know how many grains you have in your sand bank. In fact the upper chamber has been blacked out to prevent you finding out. You only know that there are a limited number and that they will all flow from top to bottom. Initially, you will probably not be too fussed by the sight of one or two grains in the bottom chamber but as the balance of the ledger shifts in favour of the lower half the perceived value of the sand in the concealed top deck will increase.

Now imagine that the rate of the sand's downward shift exactly parallels that of the passing of the days and nights of your life. (24 grains a day, for example.)

You get the picture, right?

Okay – so now replace the grains of sand with, say, gold coins. Your temporal bank account is now inexorably emptying before your very eyes at a rate of twenty four 'life dollars' a day.

Armed with such an irrefutable visual and monetary reminder you may be prompted to think *far more* strategically about how you invest your dollars. Time is literally money – it's just that it's all outgoing. Your account will not be replenished. Even your god won't pay you interest or provide you with a rolling credit facility and there is no such thing as an existential bond market. Even worse, your capital stock is being drawn upon whether you like it or not. Life, it seems, is all expenditure and no revenue.

Except that you have a choice. Not *whether* to spend but what to buy – and even though everything you purchase will ultimately be re-possessed without the possibility of appeal or recompense – you can either enjoy the shopping experience or drag yourself through life's supermarket aisles wishing you were doing something else.

I could go on extending this metaphor endlessly but I'm sure you're *au fait* enough with retail outlets and basic budgeting to have got the point by now.

By rendering the time equation in more concrete terms we can now begin to ask those big life questions with unambiguous clarity and to uncover answers that will most likely move us to live a different way.

So the next time you find yourself working hard to satisfy the whims of some petty tyrant – or you wake up wondering whether your career was worth your marriage or missing out on your daughter's childhood – consult the numbers. Is the present you are sacrificing worth the future you imagine? Sometimes it will be but a lot of the time it won't be; especially as the supply of available funds tightens and your life currency increases in relative value.

Personally, I have found that this way of framing the problem of how to balance out the competing pressures on my time has enabled me to confront fear face on – because, let's not sugar coat it, it was mostly my fear that kept me rubbing along with the same old/same old. I was afraid of being wrong. Scared that my apparent failure would be visible to others. That I would be judged foolish. Lose friends. Be poor. Miss out somehow.

Sound familiar?

Once it became clear that beneath my haughty bohemian exterior was a spirit crushing conformist fear stopping me from privately and publically embracing who I was and what I wanted … well, that fear began to evaporate. In fact, writing this book is the next chapter in my liberation struggle.

Fortunately for me – and hopefully for you – I have discovered a means of working it all out and weighing it all up. A way that refuses to let me continue in denial. A formula that reminds me in clear, numeric terms how fear, custom and vanity erode my potential for happiness. (See Chapter 2 for the maths.)

This is why I have ditched so-called spirituality and become an economist. An hourglass economist. Dedicated to the kind of wealth that can never be measured in cash or cachet, or scored in the brownie points of enlightenment. It is, instead, the richness that comes from having the guts to do whatever I want.

PS: Beware of the 'sunk cost fallacy'.

Over the last few decades we have dramatically increased our understanding of common cognitive biases, (evolved and/or subconscious neurological and perception biases that skew our thinking, slant our worldview and, significantly, affect our ability to evaluate risk). The sunk cost fallacy relates to our habit of persevering with choices, economic or otherwise, because we have already invested money, time, reputation or other resources into an objective. In other words, we routinely send good money after bad. Aside from being a budgeting faux pas, sunk cost fallacy also applies to bigger life choices. We stick with what we know (status quo bias) because we tell ourselves that having already invested so much time and effort it would 'be a shame' or 'a waste' if we switched tack, even if change is the most rational and value-positive option. Point being, sinking even more of your precious years into a misery-making lifestyle is a bad investment. Thus, it is never too late to 'let stuff go' and try a different strategy.

2.
THE DODGY MATHEMATICS OF POTENTIAL HAPPINESS

or

Weighing the inputs, measuring the output
& fixing the odds

What if we could create a simple formula for happiness
– a way for each of us to understand in clear terms
the relative impact of the forces that drive our conscious and
unconscious choice making and, in effect, shape our everyday lives?

In this chapter I utilise the economists' conceptual framework by creating my own mathematical formula for predicting happiness outcomes. Having done that, I create two fictional examples and further explore how the equation might work before showing how the 'mathematical' approach can be the start of genuinely positive life change – if we're honest.

H appiness is a condition that we all aspire to in one form or another (even if we prefer to call it joy, contentment, meaning, etc). Regardless of our semantic preference, philosophical standpoint, religious conviction or self-proclaimed level of enlightenment, every one of us can imagine a 'feeling state' called happiness (or whatever) where we would much rather be. Even if we accept that it is a largely unattainable and perhaps delusory goal – indeed, even if we don't think it *is* a goal – when we're being truthful we still catch ourselves 'striving' for it.

Cue the ten million things we've done to try and get it. Prayed, fasted, studied, shopped, worked, accumulated, competed, cheated, got high, screwed around, chased adrenalin, had surgery, had kids and so on. Sages, shrinks and self-help sorts have all tried to light our path to it. Charlatans and shonks have joined in, exploiting our unsated and often desperate hunger for it. In fact, happiness is a mega-trillion dollar industry that employs millions, chews up valuable resources and underpins every fashion disaster that ever was.

The thing is, when we throw out the confusing and contradictory plethora of 'happy pills' we are invariably drawn to one obvious conclusion. Happiness, whatever it may or may not be, comes from within. It is an attitude.

Simplistic and New Agey though that sounds, it is also true that even our *attitudes* arise and exist in a wider context – and the overriding 'wider context' is the small matter of the rest of the universe. That pesky thing called reality (cosmos, existence, etc) with which we maintain a foundational, life-long relationship.

So let's suppose that instead of relying entirely on fuzzy and hopeful spiritual/psychological fixes, we broke those attitudes down and wedded them to the clarity of mathematics? What if we could create a simple formula for happiness – a way for each of us to understand in clear terms the relative impact of the forces that drive our conscious and unconscious choice making and, in effect, shape our everyday lives?

As previously stated, the aim of this book is to get economical with normally spiritual matters – and vice versa – and so in order to stick to that heretical brief and deliver on the promise of the above I have done what the financial wizards so often do and resorted to alchemy.

Ever since the processing grunt of computers began to increase exponentially, economists and market players alike have turned to the number crunching muscle of silicon circuitry. As a result algorithms and mathematical models have proliferated. These formulae now trigger billions of stock transactions every day and frame institutional responses to market conditions.

But of course, there is an ironic lack of precision in all this maths. Indeed, the linear rigour of numbers will never be able to truly reflect the super-complexities of the economy. Human behaviour will always flummox the theorists. After all, we are all prone to making irrational choices. To being flat out wrong. We are not yet the coolly calculating robots of sci-fi lore.

However, despite knowing this, the boffins continue to wheel out their formulae, as if the mess and noise of reality could somehow be transfigured into neat numerical predictability. Just as some once hoped that lead could be turned into gold using devilishly clever jiggery-pokery.

Thus, in the spirit of economics and other magical arts, I offer you the highly dodgy, alchemical mathematics of happiness. Suffice it to say, I have arbitrarily selected the criteria, weighted the various components and fiddled the numbers in order to create what I now call the PHI, or Potential Happiness Index.

Levity notwithstanding, the PHI considers a bunch of serious practical, psychological and cultural phenomena. Chief amongst them is our old friend time. In addition it takes into account such things as social expectation, emotional states, ethics, health and wherewithal.

The guiding principle here is that by weighing up all these often conflicting forces in our lives we can arrive at a clearly quantified outcome; namely, our chance of being happy expressed as a percentage.

Whilst you can fudge the figures in order to drive your PHI north, (in fact over 100%), that's not really the point. If this exercise is to be in any way informative absolute honesty is best. Sure, it might be uncomfortable at first but I believe the process will, at the very least, encourage you to examine the drivers that shape your choices and, furthermore, help you to get a clearer picture of how the weight and importance you give to each of them affects your overall potential for future happiness. If anything, the sheer act of comparative valuation should provide a useful snapshot of where you're at, where you'd like to be and what you could do in order to get there.

And now – for the pedants and legally minded amongst you – the disclaimer.

> Though it is patently obvious to the rest of us that the following is laced with a liberal dose of tongue-in-cheek 'humour' and does not offer any guarantee, nor specifically mandate any particular course of action or inaction, nor indeed make any special claims to facilitate greater awareness, karmic pay off or general satisfaction, I would just like to say that the following does not offer any guarantee, nor specifically mandate any particular course of action or inaction, nor indeed make any special claims to facilitate greater awareness, karmic pay off or general satisfaction.

And now – having shaved off the dimwits – we may now proceed to the numbers. Or rather, the letters.

THE PHI FORMULA

NB:

Once again, before we go any further, let me assure you that this WILL NOT REQUIRE ANY MATHEMATICAL GENIUS on your part. Indeed, getting the maths right isn't really the point. The PHI is a mechanism for understanding how the various forces in your life – or the 'multi-variate inputs' if you want to get fancy – affect your happiness potential. It is simply a more formal means of focusing your attention on the comparative value you give to each of these inputs and of how they relate. The bottom line here is really this: are my habits, beliefs and subsequent actions truly working to my benefit or do they serve to weigh me down and strand me in ongoing dissatisfaction?

How can you tell that this is a serious, complex mathematical equation? Simple – because there are no numbers. All great maths is about letters and other indecipherable squiggles, is it not?

At this stage you will almost certainly have no idea what the nominated hieroglyphs stand for – apart from identifying the T shaped squiggle as being something to do with time.

So, without further ado, I present the underpinning mathematics of economic spiritualism – my flakily constructed, back-of-napkin formula for ascertaining the likelihood of future happiness.

$$PH = \frac{\frac{\left(\frac{C}{T}\right) + A + Eq}{\left(\frac{V}{R}\right) + \left(\frac{O}{E}\right)} + W}{T}$$

DECIPHERING THE PHI ALPHABET

PH: Potential Happiness – expressed as a percentage.

Given the comparative values of all the (multi-variate) inputs what are the chances of you being happy going forward?

C: Capacity – expressed as a percentage.

If 100% is perfect health and unhindered ability to do whatever you want whenever you want without your body or mental state intervening, and 0% is death, where do you find yourself? Age and other factors – buggered knees, failing eyesight, increasing agoraphobia, etc – will clearly impact this number. Although it may be difficult, if not impossible to get a truly accurate measure without a thorough medical examination, you probably have a vaguely reasonable idea of where on the capacity spectrum you sit right now.

Having arrived at that number, discount it a further 10-15%; reason being that virtually all of us tend to overestimate our capacity. (For example, I'm tempted to opt for 80% but in reality it's probably closer to 70%, if not lower.)

T: Time remaining – numbered in years.

How many good years do you think you have left? As an example – at age 53 – I have chosen 37.5. My long-lived ancestors, generally sound health and reasonably optimistic mindset have guided my choice here.

You will note that I said good years. By good I mean not the years you think you might spend cooped up in a nursing home wetting yourself. Being alive but otherwise restricted, incapacitated and fed mush by a disgruntled nurse does not, in my view, really count as living.

In addition, unforeseen circumstances can play no part in the calculation of this number – so I'm not asking you to get actuarial and factor in the minute probabilities of being murdered, run over or killed in a freak trampolining accident.

Lastly, if you're worried about tempting fate here, my advice is: a) don't be, and b) avoid trampolines.

A: Sense of Achievement – on a scale of 0-10.

Humans are busy, goal-oriented animals. We hatch plans, start projects, dream mighty dreams and fight one another to the death to make sure we win that cup, get that girl or boy or solve that age old problem. Our culture enshrines and exalts ambition as a form of sacred duty. It's why people you meet at functions invariably ask, so what do you do? Indeed, we are pretty well defined by what we do. I am a writer, etc.

Whether its bucket lists, corporate ladders or stairways to heaven we are compulsive strivers. Attainment addicts. All working towards what we're assured is success and what we hope will then become a kind of fulfilment. The huge psychological pay-off we get when we achieve these objectives makes all our struggles seem like a prudent investment strategy. We feel vindicated. Validated. Worthwhile. As though we have contributed somehow. Profited from our endeavours.

The price of dreaming, of course, is the massive downer of failure – of thwarted ambition, of less than expected results, of being overlooked, or worse, of being labelled a loser.

To exacerbate matters, even when we do succeed we are in the habit of conjuring other, more urgent goals to replace the ones we've just ticked off. In fact, most of us exist in a state of permanent (if mild) dissatisfaction. Privately, we look in the mirror and mark ourselves fairly poorly – even if we know that this is a self-defeating, socially amplified folly.

So, if 0 is abject and total failure on all fronts and 10 is the rosy glow of post-ambition success, how do you feel? Yes, feel. This number has much more to do with your perception than it does with external measures – if only because nearly all of those supposedly verifiable markers are themselves totally arbitrary and subjective.

It is worth noting here that a low (sub 5) score should, if you're being honest, drive down the next number on the list, for reasons which are about to become obvious.

Eq: Equanimity – on a scale of 0-10.

Typically defined as a sense of equilibrium, or a balanced and calm view of things – especially in times of stress and high drama – equanimity is a kind of clear-eyed acceptance. Sort of like, okay, this is how things are, in which case I'll just …

Within the frame of the PHI, equanimity is a measure of how calmly you accept your current situation, whatever it may be. For example, if you're busting your arse to change your circumstances – relationship, career, etc – and stressing hard about not getting there, then your score would be relatively low. On the other hand, if you're working towards change but accepting the various potholes, dead ends and wrong turns that confuse the path, your equanimity score would be higher. Of course, if you're totally cool with where you're at, your Eq number will be right up there.

In a nutshell, this number has to do with calmness, taking the longer view and accepting one's shortcomings with grace. As we get older, this feeling (or ability) typically increases.

V: Validation – on a scale of 0-10.

As social animals we all require a dose of external/social/cultural validation – even if we pretend we don't. This is rooted in evolution and cemented in very early childhood. As infants we look to the external for everything. Literally. Food, love, bum wiping – even the notion of I. All of this comes from the external. From parents, siblings and so on. Without the external there would be no internal.

However, as adults our relationship with the external is complicated. Our well-developed sense of identity – call it ego, if you must – begins to conflict with the messages we receive from loved ones and society more generally. Whilst we all accept the idea that kids and teens are prone to peer pressure and value social acceptance highly, most of us adults are less prepared to admit that we're still highly susceptible to the 'being included' bug. At some point we have all indulged in the defiant fantasy of the inviolable self. Fuck you! I can do whatever I want, maaaan.

The challenge with scoring the V is to be honest. Despite all your individuality rhetoric, how much do you still crave/want/seek/hope for validation from those who matter? Or even from cute strangers on buses? Indeed, to what extent do your personal and professional relationships revolve around your need for validation and how much of climbing that mountain is about being applauded for doing so?

At this stage of my life, I'm still prepared to publically confess to 2.5.

R: Relationships – on a scale of 0-10.

Most people will score this one highly. It's the social animal thing again. Humans don't just want to connect – we actually need to in order to stay alive and sane. Sure, at a basic level our DNA drives this, yet even if we take the reproductive urge out of the equation a majority of us would say that our relationships are the most important thing in our life – with the possible exception of health.

That said, relationships can be fucking annoying. Often they get tangled up with social expectation and mired in repetition and obligation. The price of keeping friends, having lovers and being in families can sometimes become prohibitive.

So, the question here is how highly do you value your relationships – and I don't just mean the sexual ones? Does that value trump ambition or mental health? Do you sacrifice personal goals for relationship security? Do you fear being alone? Hate being single?

Other valid questions here include: are relationships more important than your career, and does it matter more *what* you do or *who* you do it with?

Yet for many of us – especially women – being in culturally ordained family and class relationships are necessary for social and physical survival. This in-builds a level of pragmatic, real world value that invariably makes redundant the bourgeois niceties of post-WW2 relationship models in the West.

The point here is that not everyone has access to the range of freedoms around the in and out points of their relationships that we in the First World now take for granted. Indeed, relationships are often literally forced upon us, especially in family settings. Consider yourself fortunate if this does not apply to you.

O: Obligations – on a scale of 0-10.

We all understand the pull of duty; the way that it can both reward and enslave. At a more mundane level, the vast majority of us have obligations around work, debt and family. For some, meeting these obligations is an article of pride or a source of social status but for the rest of us they are simply tasks we are prepared to endure with a minimum of serious complaint. Though we may begrudge the grind of duty from time to time – and it may seem insufferably dull - the core problem with the big O arises when it rubs up against deeply held beliefs. When it comes into direct conflict with Ethics.

To what extent do we allow ourselves to hide behind 'but I had to'? What part of duty is merely an abdication of personal responsibility? Or fear? Or a simple lack of initiative and imagination?

Again, you might argue that this is little more than over-privileged navel gazing – especially when you take into account the billions of people around the world who still live in much stricter honour cultures than we in the West do. For these people, personal choice is a luxury, if not an unimaginable fantasy. Or indeed, an appalling decadence.

So ask yourself – how important is it for you to fulfil your mandated duties? Is it a point of honour or simply something to ping off with the minimum of effort and energy expended?

E: Ethics – on a scale of 0-10.

Before we begin, I need to clearly delineate Ethics from Obligation. Whereas the latter is more akin to simple obedience (or polite acceptance at best), moral action requires free choice in order to be considered moral. In other words, without the realistic possibility of immoral action there can be no genuinely moral action. The good must be actively chosen – not simply performed by rote or executed as a means of accruing brownie points.

Even if the moral waters are often muddy we all have a code of ethics – things we tell ourselves we would or would not do given certain circumstances. We may be morally vegan or deeply Christian, or a greenie who can't countenance the idea of contributing to the mountain of plastic in landfill. Whatever they are, most of us have belief boundaries we would rather not cross.

Yet we all find ourselves in a world that routinely confronts our cherished beliefs. Do we take that exceptionally well-paying gig with the rainforest raping mega-corp? Do we turn down the chance to have sex with that outrageously desirable and conspicuously available hottie or do we quietly regret the missed opportunity forever and a day?

It's also worth asking how much our precious ethics are really worth in the face of reality. Will we remain prisoners in a self-imposed ideological straitjacket or can we allow ourselves a little latitude? Indeed, are ethics mostly a righteous indulgence? Little more than a priggish pose?

In light of all this, what is the real value of your treasured moral narrative?

W: Wherewithal

Here is where we bow to the purely practical. Despite the current suburbanite fashion for believing that there is no real world – that everything is an emanation of self – I am of the view that in fact there is a universe which exists independent of me and my point of view. Furthermore, here on Earth in the twenty-first century, that avowedly real universe imposes certain environmental constraints on me. Some of them lay outside the locus of my control, others I am able to influence significantly.

Thus, as part of PHI, factoring in the notion of wherewithal – or functional capacity to operate in the wider world – is entirely appropriate. Access to finance and social/professional networks make a palpable difference. As do the prevailing environmental conditions – boom, bust, interest rates, legalities, war, peace, impending alien invasion and so on.

$$W = En(F+N)$$

- En: Prevailing environmental conditions – good or bad? – expressed as a percentage.
- F: Your finances – healthy or not so? – on a scale of 0-10.
- N: Your networks – useful insiders or decorative outsiders? – on a scale of 0-10.

SPELLING IT OUT

NB:

> Before commencing, please note that I have worked out PHI answers by calculating to three decimal places using the calculator on my phone. I hope that's precise enough.

The best way to illustrate the efficacy of the PHI is to resort to a little fiction. Thus, in keeping with the book's theme, I have created two case studies, both deliberately overstated and stereotypical.

1: The CEO

At the age of 45 the CEO is the epitome of apparent success. As the boss of the large and hugely profitable Evil Sludge Corporation, CEO is fabulously well remunerated, has a great reputation and plenty of friends amongst business and power elites. There's a gleaming yacht berthed in an exclusive marina, a villa on the Cote d'Azur and a ritzy upmarket apartment decorated with highly-priced original artworks. However, CEO works incredibly long hours and feels the burden of responsibility pressing hard on very stressed shoulders. Sleep is almost impossible without pills. As for family, the spouse and kids sometimes seem like strangers – afterthoughts. Mostly, they are bought off with expensive gifts. Meanwhile, CEO's diet is poor and, despite early AM gym sessions, the body is beginning to show signs of wear. Although smart enough to recognise that not everything in the garden is as rosy as it could be, CEO has decided to keep going until 50 in the hope that there will be both ample cash and enough good years left to make up for lost time.

2: The Bourgeois Buddhist

BB used to work for the Evil Sludge Corporation until the kids were born. One parental epiphany later and BB ditched the career ladder, went vego, aligned their chakras and worked assiduously to achieve a higher vibration. Next up, BB learned the art of detachment – so much so that the unvaccinated kids are now convinced that BB is too busy being enlightened to bother loving them. Meanwhile, the 'over it' ex-partner is sick of being spoken down to and listening to lectures about chem trails and getting off the grid – especially since BB appears permanently attached to the latest iGadget, despite preaching the non-material benefits of divine poverty. None of which bothers BB at 53, for BB believes that everything happens for a reason; including the lung cancer they will soon develop as a result of a furtive smoking habit.

Now imagine that CEO and BB meet up one day in the waiting room of a downtown Thai massage joint and get talking about life, the universe and the looming future. CEO casually mentions something called the Potential Happiness Index. (Apparently, an FX trader buddy raved about it one morning on the treadmills.) Inspired, or at least curious, BB promptly downloads the app onto yet another brand new wi-fi enabled smart device. Intrigued, both proceed to plug in some numbers.

	CEO	BB
Capacity	70%	80%
Time remaining	35 years	32 years
Achievement	4	7
Equanimity	5	9
Validation	7	2
Relationships	5.5	3
Obligations	8.5	2.5
Ethics	3.5	9
Wherewithal*	9.35	1.7
Environment	55%	20%
Finances	9	5
Networks	8	3.5

*as a result of $W = En(F+N)$

Of course, both are as prone to over- and underestimation as you and I. The numbers therefore are not merely subjective but highly debatable. Luckily, strict accuracy is not the point of the exercise. Rather, the aim is comparative evaluation (understanding the web of inter-relationship these powerful forces exist in). Running a mathematical rule over the various drivers that shape our choices and have an impact on our potential happiness enables us to less ambiguously assess the relative importance we give each one. To re-evaluate the value we place on stuff.

In combination, our two avatars' numbers very much reflect their varying world views and states of mind. Although the CEO feels less healthy in body and more duty bound, they maintain a measured, informed optimism about the world. Conversely, BB's cool detachment and high Equanimity number are undercut by a conspiracist's belief that the 'system is fucked' and civilisation will soon collapse.

Having run the figures to three decimal places the answers come out thus:

- CEO's PHI = 0.352 = 35.2%
- BB's PHI = 0.666 = 66.6%

The obvious question here is what does any of this mean? Is BB really almost twice as likely to be happy going forward than CEO? And anyway, isn't this all a bit arbitrary?

Indeed it is. I will not pretend otherwise. However, the point here isn't to posit a watertight proof or impose a strict new orthodoxy. Rather, this is an exercise in beginning a more serious and measured conversation about how we actually live our lives and how the ascribing of value shapes our most far reaching life choices. The PHI is a starting point model, a conversation starter, not a magic formula.

As recent advances in neuroscience have illustrated, most of our decisions – everything from grocery buying to choosing a mate – are driven unconsciously by a combination of emotional, rational and information gathering centres in the brain. Even if we don't consciously recognise it, we are constantly engaged in value judgement; assessing risk and reward using a raft of measures, including familiar dichotomies like instant pleasure versus future gain, and gratification versus guilt.

The participation of the conscious mind in all this weighing up of alternatives is, it transpires, not as significant as we might like to believe. Indeed, our evolved animal capacities and proclivities inform much of what our civilised minds decide. For example:

- The pattern loving nature of our brains – which sort and sift sense data in a highly regulated and edited fashion – thereby underpinning our tendency to rely on assumptions.
- Our hardwired kin and clan loyalties – and their ugly offshoots, racism and nationalism.
- The disgust reflex – which fuels our almost universal squeamishness around blood, shit and bugs.

For all our post-millennium sophistication we remain under the influence of primitive gravity. Not entirely dominated by it – but certainly not free of it. Hence the PHI's focus on the commonalities that affect social primates: personal and group relationships, the need for social/cultural validation, the pressures of obligation, (to abide by group norms), and the pursuit of projects and their socially underwritten esteem benefits.

In fact, drilling down, the PHI is based around a set of core beliefs about human beings – most notably that we are mortal, social animals living in a world over which we have very limited power. Furthermore, our fear of death and its associated delusion of control are the central pillars of a denialist culture that separates us from the rest of nature, from one another and from the pursuit of a genuine and sustainable happiness.

It doesn't take a genius or a conspiracy theorist to work out that in place of truly self-authored meaning and fulfilment we have wheeled in money, power, status, honour and the hubris of spiritual superiority. Even though these externally mandated predilections have their roots in the basic fact of our belonging to a mortal simian herd, they have nonetheless propelled us to create an ecologically unstable, abstract society that routinely mistakes the ownership of shiny objects for happiness and has a bewildering habit for ideological excess and genocide.

Here again we see the idea of value at play.

> **We are animals!**
>
> Though we generally use the term 'animals' to refer to non-human lifeforms on this planet, we just as routinely forget (or deny) that we too are animals. Humans are simply the current apex predator in the biosphere. We are a gendered, social, hierarchical species and the legacy of our evolved capacities and proclivities – although often unconscious and 'hidden' – remains strong in us all. What we think of as 'civilisation' is a lately adopted overlay, a form of social contract refined over millennia to better enable herd synergies and, thus, group and individual survival.

- An 'in group' member's life is more precious than the life of an 'out group' member.
- God loves people like me more than people like you.
- A princess is more valuable as a hostage than a scullery maid.
- *My* standing in the community is worth more than *your* wish to marry *that* guy.
- This year's model is more prized than last year's.
- In the long run all this overtime will be better for the kids than me spending a few wet Saturdays watching them do badly at sport.

The PHI asks us to think numerically about relative values because, perversely, despite the fact that we are almost always weighing up one thing against another, we do so in a nebulous and often self-defeating way. By neglecting to think clearly about how our valuations effect our overall wellbeing we are assigning ourselves to either wishy-washy aspirational cliché chasing or to a life spent straining at the leash of other's expectations. In a way, both are abdications.

Whilst it's obvious that mathematical hocus pocus cannot hope to magically unravel all the ambiguities or accurately resolve the unknowns we all live with, the use of a numeric/economic frame can help to shed a cleaner, clearer light on the influence of the most pervasive narratives in our lives.

And when the nominated values of all these belief commodities are measured against the value of the existential reserve currency – time – we get a much more focused and helpful picture of how we might proceed towards that thing called happiness.

AN EXERCISE IN COMPARISON

Now let's revisit our friends CEO and BB and make some adjustments to their numbers. This will allow us to see how variations in the value of their inputs influence their potential happiness outcomes. Whilst this may seem – and indeed is – idiotically obvious, the illustration of it is, well, illustrative.

You may recall mention of BB's looming lung cancer; so let's roll the clock forward past the diagnosis and imagine what might happen.

Freshly confronted by the hard-edged fact of life's fragility, BB is finding it more difficult to remain detached. The after-life narrative to which BB has clung (reincarnation) is increasingly unable to hold at bay the shudder of mortality BB feels whenever he/she coughs up blood or find him/herself a little too wheezy for comfort. Indeed, faced with an undeniable reduction in the Capacity number, BB now feels it necessary to adjust the other numbers in the PHI equation, beginning with the crucial value of T.

	BEFORE	NOW	NOTE
Capacity	80%	60%	Shortness of breath = less physical activity
Time remaining	32 years	25 years	No more smoking and no chemo + positive attitude reduces predicted overall loss
Achievement	7	5.5	Realises there are a few more things to tick off
Equanimity	9	7.5	Not quite so calm these days
Validation	2	4	Needs more reassurance – yes, you're *so* right
Relationships	3	7	Reaching out to others more – especially the kids
Obligations	2.5	4	Taking others' concerns more into consideration
Ethics	9	7	Cutting themself a bit more slack these days
Wherewithal *	1.7	1.2	* as a result of W = En(F+N)
Environment	20%	15%	System even more fucked + medicine is corrupt
Finances	5	3	Reiki sessions + new ultra-organic diet are pricey
Networks	3.5	5	Alternative health support group is a bonus
PHI	**0.666**	**0.587**	

Running the new numbers to three decimal places, we find that BB's potential for happiness has reduced from 66.6% to 58.7%, amounting to an 11.9% reduction. In other words, a 25% drop in Capacity (80% down to 60%) has only reduced the final PHI number by roughly half that amount.

However, in the above model, we've sensibly nudged all the figures roughly in accordance with how we might imagine things would fly in real life. Now let's try something a little more extreme.

Suppose that's BB's cancer diagnosis fires them up with a life changing sense of urgency, such that – despite their intellectual rejection of Western medical intervention and their underlying belief that a cleaner lifestyle will prolong their stay – they feel madly driven to tick off all those bucket list items they had previously let go of. In light of this BB scores Achievement as a mere 3 and, consequently, drops their Equanimity number to 6.

Calculated to three decimal places, this gives BB a PHI of just 44.7%. Thus, BB's reduced sense of achievement and balance has resulted in a 32.9% drop in their original happiness potential (down from 66.6% to 44.7%). What, I wonder, does this tell us about a life driven by a desire for attainment – or indeed the 'must see before you die' imperative beloved of listicle creators and lifestyle luminaries?

Meanwhile, our imaginary CEO is also contemplating the nature of ambition. Despite climbing to the top of the corporate ladder they still have a nagging sense of 'not having quite got there yet'. Within the prevailing culture of big business this tendency for restless striving and continual incremental improvement meets with the approval and admiration of colleagues, competitors and shareholders. And, like CEO, they too are prepared to forgive and/or overlook morally questionable practises if: a) they don't get caught, and b) they don't negatively impact the bottom line.

Yet when the Evil Sludge Corporation oversteps the line once too often – and innocent telegenic kiddies are affected – the CEO has an attack of guilt. Suddenly, ethics become important. Serious questions are asked about the validity of the 'profit at all costs' mentality that has fuelled CEO's wealth and success and, in turn, this prompts a re-score of the PHI inputs.

	BEFORE	NOW	NOTE
Capacity	70%	70%	Unaffected – doesn't factor in mental health
Time remaining	35 years	35 years	Unaffected – doesn't do existential crises
Achievement	4	4	Fresh new perspective balanced out by ethical downgrading of past attainments
Equanimity	5	3	Not feeling so good about self now
Validation	7	8	Needs even more reassurance – assuage guilt

	BEFORE	NOW	NOTE
Relationships	5.5	8	Suddenly, people matter more
Obligations	8.5	5	Less inclined to be such a shameless sell-out
Ethics	3.5	9	Oh god, those poor little kiddies
Wherewithal *	9.35	7.5	* as a result of $W = En(F+N)$
Environment	55%	50%	Scandal hammers stock – risk of portfolio contagion – job not so secure
Finances	9	10	Actually, I'm really fucking rich
Networks	8	5	And anyway, who are these people?
PHI	**0.352**	**0.380**	

Being a measureable results kind of person, CEO is not exactly overwhelmed by the slight uptick in the PHI. In the language of finance, they think of it in these terms: the reported 8% increase failed to meet market expectations and CEO's share price is expected to come under heavy selling pressure.

This prompts another idea. Bearing in mind that the execs of listed companies are judged by the ups and downs of the share price, the CEO switches focus to the question of Validation. As a result, they arrive at the realisation that so much of their life and work – and indeed Evil Sludge's chances of recovering from the cute kiddy scandal – revolves around impressing others. Upon creating and maintaining positive beliefs in the market about success, character and credit worthiness.

As someone used to number crunching and mathematical modelling, they decide to run a quick test and drop their V score from 8 to 4. A few keystrokes later and the formula comes back with 0.458 – or 45.8% – thereby resulting in a healthy looking 30.1% increase in potential happiness (up from 35.2%).

However, with the PHI still sitting under 50%, CEO turns their gaze to Validation's cousin, Obligation, reasoning that both revolve around meeting expectation. A subsequent drop in the O number from 5 to 3 results in a revised PHI of 0.523, which equates to a 52.3% chance of happiness across the forecast period.

The challenge for CEO over the medium-long term is how to implement the changes – turning newfound *awareness* into practical, lasting reform.

THE TAKE OUTS

Okay, so what's the deal with all this semi-facetious, pseudo mathematical pondering? What has this really shown us?

To answer that question, I will seek recourse to autobiography. Like so many of us in the materially privileged post-WW2 West, I have had the advantage of living in an era of decreasing violence, (despite what the tabloid media keeps trying to tell me).

What's more, historically high social mobility, (I'm a working class outer suburban kid with a taxpayer-funded Uni degree), and increasingly liberal social attitudes have allowed me to choose the life of a freelance bohemian with almost no blowback. As my dad likes to say, I am amongst history's winners – and indeed, I do daily give thanks for my incredible good fortune in this regard.

However, I have to be honest and say that I have not been particularly happy in my life. Sure, there's a complex back story to this – a web of proclivity, circumstance, poor choice and aesthetic preference – but that's not the focus of this exercise. My intention here is to outline a forward looking mode of *thinking about* and *strategising around* that fact. Not an ideology or utopian project. Not a shiny new bauble or groovy underground drug habit. Nor even a higher vibration. Just a frame of analysis.

Having done everything from the sensible marriage/ job/house routine to the esoteric Reiki channelling trip, and even the repulsive reductionism of the 'self as a brand' cult, I woke up after the requisite whitefella mid-life crisis to find myself well and truly over the isms and not at all convinced by any of the standard cookie cutter narratives so beloved of virtually everyone I knew (God, destiny, enlightenment, etc).

It was time for a little spiritual minimalism – for a good hard look at the real core of things. What really mattered to me, what was of genuine value and what was just habit, or worse, self-important delusion and hubris?

Naturally I had some pretty sound instincts about what the answers would be but it was only when I changed the very architecture of the analysis, the tools of investigation, that the 'problem' could even be stated – let alone solved – in a useful fashion.

My PHI score

Of course, it would be remiss of me to rely purely on fictional examples, so here are my numbers. What they tell me, more than anything else, is that my current portfolio of beliefs and behaviours appear quite likely to deliver ongoing happiness dividends – which, at this point in my life, I will take as a definite win.

Here then is my PHI scorecard:

Capacity:	75%
Time left:	37.5yrs
Achievement	9
Equanimity:	7.5
Validation:	2.5
Relationships:	5
Obligations:	1.5
Ethics:	3.5
Wherewithal:*	4.5

* as a result of $W = En(F+N)$

Environment:	60%
Finances:	5.5
Networks:	2

In conclusion, my PHI number is 0.65104, which then translates as a 65.104% chance of sustainable happiness going forward.

NB: To find out more, and to drill further into the subsoil of my persona, go to Appendix 2.

And that's what the PHI is truly about. Choosing a language. Framing an approach. Using Occam's razor to strip back the ideological, quasi-religious clutter of self-help, spirituality and the search for meaning; then replacing it with a simple, pragmatic means of examining the life-shaping *relationship* between the fundamental universals that play into our happiness or lack thereof.

The PHI is a start point. A neat, arithmetically encapsulated way of sifting, sorting and re-pricing stock on the existential equity exchange – remembering that just as it is in the money economy, so too it is in your personal marketplace, where the fluctuating price of the various stocks are related in a complex web of perceived value and broader expectations about future market moves.

You can use the PHI to run models. Test out the effects of different numbers. Arrive at a desirable equilibrium – one that gives you an existential investment strategy that delivers the kind of happiness dividend you're after.

Of course you can try out highly unlikely combinations and arrive at a grossly inflated and unrealistic PHI score but this will likely end in the same way as most overly optimistic high risk market positions. Badly.

Your challenge – as it was for me – is to be honest. Dodgy maths can only go so far and metaphors drawn from economics will soon grow tired. If anything, this exercise is about creating a platform for honesty. By stripping away moral judgement and mandated end-points, it allows us to ponder the importance we place on certain things and how this assigning of value impacts our overall sense of wellbeing.

And, of course, it does all this in the context of a real world – rather than an imagined or desired one. It places all of our introspective weighing up in time and society, in a web of relationship. In what remains of our lives.

3.

THE ATTAINMENT FETISH

or

The gimp mask of bigger better bucket lists

It's easy to see how sado-masochistic our commoditised,
fetishised achievement cult has become. In the dungeon of
incessant striving, the doms and subs whip one another into
a frenzied cycle of fleeting success and ritual humiliation.

In this chapter, I outline the reasons to get off the socially engineered attainment treadmill. In addition, I suggest that by abandoning externally mandated life meanings and refusing to be drawn into the fetish of achievement and judgement so beloved of marketing types and self-improvement fascists, we can truly write the story of our own lives.

A recent beer ad underscored the point, neatly encapsulating the fact that the competitive cult of cachet has wormed its way deep into our private lives. Are you an experience collector? it asked its audience.

Of course the unspoken assumptions behind the question are far more interesting than any of the possible answers. 'Collecting' cool experiences, ticking them off a to-do list, is equated not only with a sense of wellbeing and achievement but will – when combined with the responsible consumption of the nominated supermarket beer brand – lead you towards a better life and therefore make you that much sexier.

This is advertising at its cynical, manipulative best. It's a pitch to our restive yearning for achievement and the gnawing insecurity and need for validation that helps fuel it. The basic message is: if you're the kind who won't settle, who climbs mountains, visits exotic locales and ruggedly adventures, (as opposed to sitting at home watching beer ads on TV), then you're our kinda guy. You're gonna stand out from the crowd. Babes are gonna love ya. And when Jimi Hendrix asks 'are you experienced?' you'll be able to say, 'sure, man' – but in a totally straight, non homo-erotic way, of course.

However, the migration of the attainment mantra from the public and professional to the private and psychological is not exactly new. Neither is it purely the result of global capitalism and liberal individualism. Indeed, history is replete with pre-industrial examples of relentless ambition. What's more, you could well argue that our mania for achievement was cemented in place by the evolutionary and environmental imperatives that drove our nomadic forebears to make tools, devise clever hunting strategies and coalesce in social/hierarchical groups. In the uncertain, dangerous and competitive world of ancient Africa it paid to get busy – and to do so en masse.

Yet, sometime after our ancestors battled their way to the top of the food chain, the arrow head of human social endeavour evolved from the spear tip of immediate protein provision to the sharpened blade of power struggles and the garnering of prestige. With the advent of the Agricultural Revolution natural shocks became ever more manageable and human society went from an aggregation of small, inter-related tribal groups fused together by concrete personal and environmental relationships to a world of larger impersonal conglomerates (super-polities) unified by increasingly abstract group identifiers and held together by frequently opaque and distant authority.

As Soviet ideologues may once have put it, working people living in these proto-states would not have had 'the bourgeois luxury of a private life'. (Or at least, not one that we in the post-modern West would recognise.) For them, achievement would most likely have revolved around socially visible and easily measureable objectives – big house, expensive objects, lots of healthy kids, plenty of provisions for the winter, etc. Spiritual, philosophical and psychological attainments would have been relegated to the realm of invisible private musing, or to the socially ordained adherence rituals of religion and fealty.

Although aristocrats and cloistered intellectuals have enjoyed the riches of individuality for millennia, the emergence of the fully fledged private life as a broad-based phenomenon is relatively recent; coming on the back of increased wealth, improved technology and the greater awareness afforded to us by advances in our understanding of mental health. These, allied with socio-economic developments like weekends, annual leave and readily available credit, have created the social space, personal time and economic conditions for a far greater range of individual 'life choices' than ever before.

Cynics and conspiracists would contend that all this so-called choice is simply the result of a creeping corporate takeover, a commodification of experience engineered by the captains of capitalism to put a price point on our most private yearnings. The aforementioned beer ad is a good example. A life enriched by great experiences can be augmented – even mediated – by your purchase of the appropriately branded beer. In this world, the right six-pack is a gateway drug to a full and rewarding life.

If the emotional manipulation stopped there the edge of it would be blunt – a stupid conflation easily undone – but the ad creatives know that for lasting effect they need to somehow suggest a social pay-off for your private choices. Just as on Facebook, where we all publically promote ourselves as the leaders of really cool and exemplary lives, so too the brand bullshitters want us to associate

---

The 'abstraction' of clan identity

There is a step-change difference between the small, blood-tied clan clusters we initially evolved to live in and the much larger, super-tribal societies we developed to replace them after the revolutions of agricultural surplus and animal husbandry. As soon as townships and cities began to form, a proto-state emerged, and – once the concrete ties of personal inter-dependence that bound our pre-Ag forebears together became unworkable when scaled up to the newer, larger population networks – a degree of abstraction, (or de-individuation and 'class' stratification), started to emerge and solidify. The focus of clan identity then shifted from our small scale and concrete personal/territorial relationships with extended family and the local environment to the less immediate, more theoretical realms of city states, ethnicity narratives and religious affiliations. Indeed, in many ways, this new 'political' identity is an early form of de-humanisation. By associating the worth of individuals with externally visible markers, like states and gods, and then marrying that to supposedly moral assertions, we effectively created the core us/them platform that underpins the childish essentialisations that operate in everything from blatant racism to polemic identity politics.

NB: For more on this theme, check out 'The Nature Problem' in Appendix 1.

purchasing choices with status, sexiness and grand statements of self-expression.

It's no longer good enough to have the biggest pay packet or the most fertile spouse, you're meant to have the most amazingest, awesomest life ever; a life so dense with astounding experiences that your friends will feel that their own paltry existences just don't measure up. In the dream world of the twenty-first century we're all stars. We can *all* achieve greatness.

And how? Because in the lottery of global capitalism everyone can be fooled into believing they're a winner. (Well, almost everyone.)

But before we convince ourselves that this is all an evil magic dreamt up by conniving central bankers or agents of the Illuminati, we should remind ourselves that the success of the bucket list philosophy is rooted in something far more fundamental than boardroom plots and ad campaigns. Even the much vaunted Protestant work ethic is underpinned by the evolutionary fact of the busy human animal. Indeed, we frequently self-identify in terms of what we *do*. Our projects (work, hobbies, spiritual quests, etc.) publically denominate us as writers, plumbers or acrobats and in turn these activities then become integral to what we think of as *our purpose*. Witness the New Agers and their 'this is what I'm here for' rhetoric, or the apocalypse-loving fundamentalists working hard to herald the end of days with suicide bombs and gory online videos. Extreme and absurd as both these narratives may be they point to the psychological truth behind sayings like 'the Devil makes work for idle hands to do'. We need to do stuff, complete things, in order to stay truly sane and functional. And, to some extent at least, we need to do so in society. We need others to notice our achievements.

The successful conquest of private life by the marketing mavens is not so much the result of a fiendishly clever mega-conspiracy but rather of a more ruthlessly targetted and successful attempt to exploit our natural tendencies.

The current amplification of this phenomenon is being powered by the internet; particularly the self-reflecting silos of social media. You Tube, Facebook and Instagram have unleashed a tsunami of show & tell. Contrast & compare was never so easy – or so instant. The online ubiquity of self-promotion (and its other half, judgement) is simply proof writ digitally that we are competitive achievement junkies vying for favourable attention from other members of the herd.

Yet whereas achievement used to be limited principally to the external, it has now moved indoors. Today, the *quality of your life* has become a socially measureable mode of attainment. Happy, healthy and wise are now points to be scored. As one recent Facebook meme declared: *self-improvement is the new sexy*.

Of course, what the new sexy brand fascists will never tell you is that if your life can be a stellar success it can also be an epic fail. Imagine the horror of being on your death bed and thinking that your very *life* was not up to scratch. That you had *failed* at existence. Not travelled enough. Not shagged enough. Not had a sufficiently deep and meaningful epiphany that made neat sense of the whole messy shebang. Or, God forbid, you got nowhere near enough Likes and Shares.

In this light it's easy to see how sado-masochistic our commoditised, fetishised achievement cult has become. In the dungeon of incessant striving, the doms and subs whip one another into a frenzied cycle of fleeting success and ritual humiliation.

But surely, you protest, there's a way for me to ease off the sweaty gimp mask of submission and battle my way into the cleansing, clear eyed light of the morning?

Why yes, of course there is – but you might not get many Likes.

THE OILY LADDER DILEMMA

The humble ladder provides us with a powerful metaphor. All those steps going up. All those rungs leading down. However, the problem with career and social ladders is that they are pyramid shaped, with access to the higher rungs severely restricted. In addition, not everyone starts at the bottom; so the universal climb-a-thon is far from fair. Furthermore, the person on the ground charged with holding the ladder steady is in fact shaking the shit out of it, such that the rain of falling climbers is more akin to a monsoon downpour than a gentle evening sprinkle.

Complicating matters is the fact that the rungs are coated with an invisible smear of oil – but not just any oil. No no, this is emotionally savvy oil. So clever in fact that it will be either sluggishly sticky or skittishly slick according to your mood. If you're feeling frustrated by your lack of upward movement it will act like glue, holding you in position and seriously hampering your progress. If, on the other hand, you have scaled the heights and are now feeling the vertigo of ennui or exhaustion – or more tellingly, the altitude sickness of having wasted so much time on so vain a pursuit – then you will struggle to hold on. Only those who are satisfied with the rung they're on or aren't stressed by up/down movement are free to ascend or descend without the threat of greasy hands. Or indeed, they can choose to skip the ladder entirely.

Because the ladder's Achilles' heel is that it needs you to believe in better. In more. In brand spanking new.

Indeed, it is nothing without your faith in progress or your fear of failure. It requires your ambition, your goal-oriented determination to meet your KPIs, tick the requisite boxes and reap the financial, social and personal rewards of achievement.

Even if your dream is to destroy the ladder.

Luckily for the ladder makers there is an almost universally accepted inevitability narrative to help stave off potential revolution and prop up the status quo. From the stoic, defeatist pragmatism of the toiling masses to the system blaming histrionics of those who would assure you that the masses only toil because evil people put fluoride in their drinking water, there are countless variations on the notion that:

- It's just the way it is.
- You gotta be real about things, right?
- Dream on, kiddo – things ain't about to change.
- Fuck, what did you expect?
- The system is rigged, man.

Whilst it's fairly clear to most of us that we live in a non-ideal world rife with inequality, injustice and poorly thought out imperatives, there is nothing inevitable about it. Highly likely given past performance, sure – but nothing like a 100% boxed up and done deal. Cultural, economic and psychological pressures notwithstanding, the lure of the ladder *can* be resisted.

As I suggested in the first two chapters, re-examining your perceptions around value is a great practical start point. However, the trick is to adopt the master's language (so to speak) and get cold and economical with your existential valuations. Furthermore, once you accept the fairly reasonable idea that your most valuable asset is time then you can take a fresh look at the relative worth of achievement.

Of course, none of this will be new to you. Most of us over forty have already worked out that the majority of our so-called achievements deliver little more than a sugar hit and ultimately leave a kind of empty aftertaste. Sometimes this manifests as regret or disappointment but more often it's like *yeah, so*. Or even, *shit, why the hell did I bother with that?* Our so-called successes turn out to be pretty underwhelming most times – like Christmas presents when you're a kid. Great for a day, then … collecting dust.

Thus it is, with advancing years, that the thought of ploughing yet more time into the pursuit of status, success or grand visions seems increasingly tiring and pointless.

Given that you already know that most of what you strive for has no real or far-reaching value and ultimately won't really deliver soul deep happiness, the obvious next question is: why bother?

However, rather than ask this question in a petulant or jaded way – like some bored teen or bitter old bastard – let's ask it in the spirit of honest inquiry. In the light of your rapidly approaching and inevitable death and in the face of a largely oblivious, uncaring and sometimes even dismissive world, why bother indeed?

Take this book, for example. I could be having an afternoon nap right now or eating the second half of the delicious patisserie item that waits alluringly in my kitchen. Christ, I could even be doing internet porn. Or almost anything but sitting in the corner of my bedroom typing this menopausal scree onto a clunky old laptop.

Without wishing to seem doomful or dramatic, here's the stark reality about this book. According to any externally measurable criteria this endeavour is almost certain to fail. Taking into account the dismal probabilities associated with 'unknowns' like me writing books, and a few persistent personal proclivities, the terrain looks roughly like this:

- This book is almost certain *not* to get published.
- If published, it is almost certain *not* to sell in significant numbers.
- If read, even loved, it is unlikely to herald a new dawn or mass reappraisal of current socio-economic norms.

+

- I almost certainly won't make any money out of if.
- I almost certainly won't get famous as a result of it.
- Sexy people won't suddenly start liking me (dammit).

+

- There is at least a 50% chance that I will get to the end and decide that this really isn't so clever and amusing after all – or even that I've changed my mind entirely.

Yet plainly, evidence notwithstanding, I *am* still bothering. Whilst my absurdly resilient optimism and the comfortably hermetic habit of writing provide *some* of the impetus for continuing – not to mention the fact that I don't have a real job and therefore have the time and mental energy for such ridiculous pursuits – I shall persist in this quixotic ramble because the real payoff isn't external. It's private. Emotional. It has something to do with my sense of myself – with what kind of person I am and wish to be. There's also the thrill of getting your ideas in order and the promise of the clarity it entails. And yes, it's kinda fun because, I'll be honest with you, I like the sound of my own voice. The sight of my own vision. The lovely glow I get when I finish these avowedly self-indulgent projects. This is why I am investing the non-renewable asset of my hours into a book of crackpot psycho-economical, existential pontification.

Now that we're clear about that, let's get back to our metaphoric ladder.

Although obvious that the ladder described above is an externality – that is, public, socially visible, etc – it only gets truly treacherous when it becomes *in*ternal. In other words, when we take it on. When we use it to compare ourselves to others. To judge them and ourselves. To provide an excuse to ignore and/or medicate our ills in a blur of ceaseless striving. To subvert our ethical beliefs to the graven image of success or undermine our closest relationships by putting them in the queue *behind* the gig, the goal or the glittering prize.

Yet, as social primates we have a hardwired need for a least a modicum of external validation, if not loads of it. For despite what the sexy new self-improvement Nazis tell us, we are *not* entirely self-contained. All of us live and form our identity in *a world* – and as such that world is our stage, our anchor and our existential GPS. Thus, the internal and the external are locked in a lifelong feedback loop. No wonder so much of our ambition and purpose are played out in public. Indeed, our culture only really rewards socially visible achievements – and insofar as it rewards private ones it only does so by forcing them out of doors. (Are you an experience collector, by any chance? Is your new improved self seriously sexy enough?)

The problem for you and I then is how to disempower the ladder; or at least not to get too thoroughly smeared with that pesky mood monitoring oil and, as a by-product, consign ourselves to plod painfully nowhere or plunge precipitously towards ignominy, irrelevance and invisibility.

However, rather than resort to the stock standard vagaries and affirmations of self-help books, life coaches and spiritual advisors, we can turn to economics. Or, more particularly, to the conceptual toolkit of economics and its power to help us measure risk, reward and value.

In the previous chapter I introduced the PHI – Potential Happiness Index – and described its purpose as creating a methodology for sifting out and comparatively weighting the importance of various human universals. Amongst these were life expectancy, relationships, ethics, financial capacity and sense of achievement. By employing some very basic arithmetic it's easy to see how a low sense of achievement number can result in a reduced probability of happiness. Moreover, the equation allows us to understand achievement in relationship with things like health, the need for validation and the pull of obligation.

Ah c'mon, you're saying, this all sounds too simple, Paulie.

Well yeah, that's the idea. To demystify. To strip away ideological narrative. To render the problem amoral. To wrench possible solutions from the clutches of external authority figures (gods, gurus, grandmas, etc) and put them firmly within our scope of our control.

What I'm most definitely *not* doing here is suggesting that coming to terms with ambition is an act of 'enlightenment' – because the bitch about enlightenment (or self-improvement) is that it's just another item on a bucket list. Fuck, it's even supposed to be sexy these days. If your goal is to reach a plateau of Zen calm but you cuss yourself for falling short, back sliding or failing to vibrate at a sufficiently high frequency, then you are simply stranded on that damn ladder. Worse, the attainment fetish will have entered your very soul. The marketing demons will have injected their reductionist, dehumanising poison into your veins and you will have become an even more hardcore achievement junkie.

Our intention here is not simply to transcend ambition or retire to a supine life of aimless drifting but to get a clearer picture of how our desire to strive and achieve affects our overall happiness. Perhaps the cleanest way of stating it is:

- How are your various projects contributing to or reducing your sense of wellbeing?
- Is your unfulfilled ambition eating your insides out?
- Do you punish yourself and/or those you love for life's almost inevitable delays, wrong turns and defeats?
- Are you ever really satisfied with where you're at ambition-wise?
- Do you look across at others and envy their spot on the ladder?
- To what extent does 'fomo' (the fear of missing out) drive you?

Whilst these are all quite complex and profound questions, I have personally found it useful to borrow the stripped back, utility driven architecture of economics to reframe the issue in simpler risk/reward terms.

Given that we are spending our life currency (time) on pursuing ambition, are the risks worth the predicted rewards? And indeed, what *are* these imagined rewards? Money? Power? Status? Or just the thrill of it all? Or maybe even the admiration of hot men? Ultimately, when we're honest about the value of the rewards we can better calculate the price of the risk.

> **The object of desire**
>
> I have found it useful to drill into my desires, to unpack my ambitions and objectives in order to better understand what I'm *really* looking for. In nearly all cases that don't involve issues of raw physical survival, it boils down to a 'feeling state'. So, not the fame and acclaim of authorship but the way that writing this book helps me feel now; which, is really good about myself and the life I'm living. In other words, the bottom line dividend arising from my investment of non-refundable time into this project (and others) is rooted in feelings of worth, freedom and ongoing self-authored purpose. The banal yet powerful distinction between 'trophy' and 'feeling that trophy engenders' can help us to disentangle socially received meanings and objectives from our own, authentic yearnings – if only because the nominated trophy (achievement) is just a place-holder for the deeper feeling state that is the *real* bedrock object of desire. Therefore, the next time you think 'oh if only I had *that* gizmo' ask yourself how it is you imagine said trinket will help you feel and if there might not be other (quicker, easier, less costly) ways to get there.

So, if you ask yourself just one question, try something like: how much is a year of my life worth? As you get older the value of that year will surely rise – and the comparative worth of the badges and trinkets of success will evaporate.

Yeah, I *know* this, you're telling me. Of course you do. We all do. Yet still we find ourselves struggling on the ladder, competing with ourselves and others to attain this goal and that objective. And just like the leather-clad denizens in the fetish bar, we wax between pleasure and pain, elation and agony, mastery and slavery.

In the final analysis, the trick is not to care – because not buying into the competitive drama of achievement dissolves its unreasonable hold over us. We can still start and complete our various projects, still be productive, still make a contribution if we choose, but we can do so without all too common 'have to' narratives and their crude pass/fail criteria hanging over our heads.

Before that though we have to find a way to not care; a way that isn't just an alternative ladder or yet another bauble of middle class wisdom status. Cue …

THE TEN MILLION THINGS YOU ABSOLUTELY DON'T NEED TO BOTHER WITH BEFORE YOU DIE

We've all seen the listicles, advice columns and ponderous books telling us we will die with a ravaging sense of incompleteness unless we visit this pristine beach, read that classic book, learn this obscure but meltingly sexy language or drop those stubborn pounds. Over the last few years the number of things we supposedly 'must' do/see/have or become has risen exponentially. Makes you wonder where any of us are supposed to find the time for all these musts.

The most intriguing aspect of the listicle life is just that – the 'must' bit. *Oh really, why must I?* What exactly will having myself photographed grinning inanely at Machu Pichu do for me? Will owning a copy of My Bloody Valentine's remastered *Loveless* album (on heavy duty German vinyl, of course), really help potential soulmates identify me in a crowd of balding Coldplay fans?

For just as it is with the 'experience collecting' lager ads, so too it is with 'before you die' lists. Beneath the obvious call to action is the deeper lure – the promise of approval. Because *doing* all this cool stuff makes us better, more believable, infinitely more fuckable people.

Of course we know that none of that is actually true. (Money can't buy you love, right?) However, the problem isn't that we don't *know* this, it's that we don't *do* anything about it. Or rather, believe that we *can't*. We may have tried previously and failed dismally, or we may find ourselves living in the clutches an honour culture that makes 'being true to yourself' a much bigger social, financial and physical risk than it would otherwise be for a happily freelance, Anglo-Saxon bohemian like yours truly. Whatever the particulars, the weight of the accumulated evidence suggests that, as a species and as a society, we are manifestly unable to wrench ourselves away from the idea that the path to a deeper happiness involves the successful doing, getting and winning of stuff. Bigger, better bucket lists for everyone!

Which loosely translates as: *more, more, more.*

And all of it played out against the backdrop of time. *Your* time. Less, less, less.

Typically, we attack these kinds of existential conundrums with either command and control mechanisms – god, king or custom – or with the softer but no less ideological frame of spiritual philosophy. One is a monopoly, the other a confuse-opoly. Both disempower their victims by making them dependent on external validation sources. Ticks of approval are transmitted through everything from obedience rituals to destiny and afterlife narratives and are disseminated via the agency of the numerous meta-ordained meanings and higher purposes that infuse every spiritual tradition from paganism to pan-theism. *I know I'm right because the higher authority says I am. Because it is written.*

In this frame, life is understood as an exercise in executing a pre-existing plan or passing a series of tests. The living are just the marionettes of destiny; either that or the unsuspecting recruits in a brutal, never ending bootcamp of conscious existence toiling their way towards Olympic quality nirvana. And all according to an imposed order, albeit a karmically benign and divinely guided one.

I regard this as a fundamentally disempowering notion. If my time is to be spent pursuing pre-ordained objectives or satisfying the assessment criteria of karma committees and didactic deities, well I'm sorry but I quit. My continued servicing of these apparently essential objectives will simply condemn me to a repetitive, ladder-locked existence – a life in which I give away my power to invisible external forces like god, destiny and social approbation in return for rewards which I already know aren't that rewarding.

To boil it down: any value or meaning in my life is *not* dependent on external authorisation to underwrite it. Divine, legal, social or otherwise.

Okay, so while that's an easily bullish thing to write, the practical reality confronting almost all of us is somewhat more entangled. We are all enmeshed in relations of mutual inter-dependence, whilst some of us find ourselves in situations of flat out financial dependence or, worse, imprisoned by actual or implied violence. These are very real considerations and I am in no way seeking to minimise or shrug off their significance. However, what I am suggesting is that, when you really drill into it, there is no 'have to'.

When you can honestly defuse the power of the countless compulsion narratives that exist in our culture you will experience a deep sense of liberation. Gandhi understood the incredible power of non-participation – and so can we all. If you choose to, you too can unleash a kind of private *Satyagraha* (truth force) on the cult of 'gotta do' and the citadel of 'must have'.

Which is where we come back to the arrow of time. Devoid of personal qualities, moral agendas or the need to be venerated, time acts universally and in a strictly egalitarian fashion; at least as we experience it as human beings. As far as time is concerned, no interest will be paid into your temporal account for good character or in recognition of sterling achievement, nor indeed to honour your fabulous collection of experiences. The electro-chemical event that is your physical life will unfold and yield to entropy regardless of whether you've climbed Everest, discovered the key to cosmic oneness or just lounged about in the tropics taking barefoot beach walks.

Time doesn't give a fuck about you and your victories. Or your sexy new improved self. Or even your persistent shortcomings. Time is not a judge.

Thus, once we come to understand time in raw currency terms – as a constant expenditure item – we effectively generate an alternative and highly practical external value measure against which to plot everything else. Rather than a needy god or entrenched social custom we are left with a blind, even-handed externality that sits beyond the self-serving manipulation of ideology and which requires nothing of us; except perhaps that we take note of its passing and, thus, of its increasing value.

In the face of this implacable certainty (mortality) almost everything else seems a little inconsequential. Even the most exquisite, expensive and expertly assembled clock in the cosmos won't stop the seconds ticking down. Won't stop you ending up where it all began. On the edge of nothing.

Therefore, since you are *spending your time* competing on corporate ladders or completing the bucket list, you are, in effect, trading non-refundable chunks of your *life* in return for … ?

When you start to view 'the attainment thing' through this prism it begins to seem much more like a fetish activity, one where the guilty little pleasures are frequently served up with lashings of ritual yet perversely acceptable pain. In addition, since time delivers exactly the same outcome to the gormless as it does to the guru, the net advantage that will accrue to you for all your competitive achieving of stuff is, well, zero.

By reminding ourselves that we are all equal in the eye of time (not to mention infinitesimally tiny) our perspective on what is important shifts. The endless competitions – for fertile mates, social status, moral high ground, etc – are understood afresh as the ultimately meaningless froth and bubble games that they truly are; and in this light the constant nagging voice urging us to achieve is left with hardly anything worth saying.

Now that we have divested the ladder of its oily power by undermining ubiquitous external ordination arguments and accepting how truly empty the supposed rewards of compliance are, we are free to discover entirely private sources of motivation. Or, to carry on the finance metaphor a little further, we can launch a private equity takeover of ambition and take a mix of both long and short positions in the personal meaning markets.

Since all such investments will require the non-refundable capital outlay of your existential reserve currency (time) it's only prudent to do some due diligence and ask: exactly *what* the fuck am I buying into here?

Under such a withering spotlight the standard issue, socially received imperatives we have structured our culture around will have their authority drastically diminished. Now all of a sudden you don't *have* to spend a fortnight trekking in Bhutan in order to seem like the kinda person with whom all self-respecting members of the appropriate gender will want to make babies. In fact, you no longer have to do anything, go anywhere or be anyone. And you will receive a signed note – on ethically sourced, fair trade, recycled, fully biodegradable hemp paper – excusing you from all future enlightenment classes.

THE REVOLUTION WILL BE POINTLESS

Now that we've decided not to bother with the endless list of things to knock off before we die, the pertinent question is: how do we fill the vacuum left behind by dethroned gods and outmoded, bourgeois, self-improvement activities?

There is a school of thought that suggests that, stripped of the supporting edifice of culture, we would all collapse into a lazy, anti-social fog of loneliness, disorientation and consuming misery. Whilst it is true that we have evolved as social primates and that, moreover, we are *fundamentally* social beings, it is also clear that rigid adherence to group norms comes at a devastating emotional, intellectual and societal cost. A price that far too many of us are still paying.

Forms of group participation predicated on custom, adherence and fear eventually reveal themselves to be hollow; little more than ritualistic re-enactments of designated inclusion behaviours. A meal ticket. Until you get sick of the junk food, that is.

- Trouble is, you gotta keep eating it.
- Not forever …
- Just until …

Of course, it is in that very space – the one between mere awareness and actual change – where denial, desperation and dishonesty coalesce to fuel and sustain our dramas, our addictions and our control mechanisms, and where we hone the habit of passive consumption; such that a highly abstract and far from perfect social environment can seem as though it were the natural order of things. *It's just how it is, right? Gotta rub along, ain't yer?*

Our evolved tendency for busy-ness, our innate sociability and a deep desire for meaning work neatly together in this instance, driving both our will and our capacity to make and execute plans. They inspire the personal and shared narratives necessary to underpin all personal projects and life meanings; in addition to fuelling cultural forms like religion, philosophy and politics.

However, as the persistence of cruelty, inequality and unsustainable convenience amply illustrate, the busy rubbing along model has delivered a mixed legacy. Whereas social order, the rule of law and a reliable measure of communal harmony are clearly shared assets, over-consumption, ravaging the environment and 'kicking the dog' are akin to acting out behaviours; the signs of a society whose individual members are either blindly or begrudgingly conceding defeat to what they believe is 'the system'. Whilst some of us undoubtedly gain from the status quo, the rest of us appear to be conducting and orienting our lives as though there were *no other viable way* of doing so. We tacitly acquiesce with a plan which, in brutally simple terms, stipulates that in return for sometimes being allowed to do what we want, we will be required to spend the rest of our lives rubbing.

Which is exactly what you would expect from a busy making, social animal who wants to make sense of everything – and be recognised and approved of for doing so.

So, the bottom line problem isn't so much that we are predisposed to operating in a competitive public arena of achievement-based striving and social judgement (of which the work environment is a prime example), it's the reasons we each *individually* chose to.

For even blind capitulation is a form of choosing. So ask yourself:

- What is the nature of my private bargain with the ladder?
- Why do I continue investing chunks of my life in pursuits that don't serve me?
- Surely it's not just habit?
- Or am I just reflexively afraid to seriously consider the alternatives?
- Or maybe I really do believe that the latest and greatest will make me happy.

Go on, be honest. It's okay – no one's watching.

However you responded to the above, please be aware that once you adapt to life without the convenience of divinities or the supporting framework of externally ordained meaning narratives, you will be free to insert your own meanings into the existential space. To re-negotiate the ladder relationship on your terms.

And your trump card is time. The ultimate unit of value. For time is literally what we are. Life is an event. A self ordering sequence of happenings in a homeostatic system. Conscious energy in constant motion. And every word in this sentence is costing you – just as every keystroke was paid directly out of my ever dwindling existential holding account.

Since our lives are *made* of time and motion, we are literally sacrificing little pieces of our life by adhering either passively or under protest to cultural and economic norms; when we live in a manner that we do not truly believe in.

So how many minutes of your allotted hour would you be prepared to wager for your chance to win the various shiny trophies of attainment? Trophies which, by the way, you will *not* be able to take with you. Glamour that will fade. History that will forget.

However, the moment we come to value something else more highly than any of the prizes currently on offer in achievement land, the crude ladder scurry of participating in the bustling ant parade is stripped of its necessity. Participation then becomes a matter of choice – and consequently we lose the 'had to' excuse.

As for reinventing motivation after the death of the usual external ordination model, moving the focus 'internal' is the key. By using the economist's conceptual toolkit to re-frame everything in relation to time and to better understand the comparative values of the various physical, psychological and social drivers of choice making, we can open up the very real possibility of choosing a life we actually *want* as opposed to the one we think we more or less *have* to live.

Suffice it to say, the nature of all these freshly minted internal positive motivations will be entirely personal and particular. However, understanding that nothing is compulsory – not even staying alive – and that no form of attainment, even those inspired by idiosyncratic purposes, will prevent your death or ensure everlasting happiness (let alone control the responses of other herd members) is pivotal. This will underwrite your long term freedom from the 'must' culture of ladder climbing, gimp-masked achievement drones – even if you *do* go to the occasional dungeon club.

After all, attainment is not a bad thing. Empty and ultimately little more than pointless vanity, yes – but not necessarily evil.

In fact, the very pointlessness of achievement is its saving grace. In a space without externally mandated meanings – without resort to the handy, higher authority get out clause – we are free to act in accordance with our own private narratives. To suggest, in the absence of pre-ordained purposes, other reasons for doing stuff. To invest our temporal capital in projects that will deliver a dividend in happiness. Not necessarily wisdom – for wisdom is too often a conceit – but in the lasting sense of being who you wish to be and of truly doing what you want.

Pointlessness is nothing less than freedom. A space awaiting a point. Others will try to get you to insert theirs. You can do so if you wish. Or you can insert your own. Both will involve costs and benefits. Both will be billed in time. But which point would *you* prefer? God's, the village elder's, the cute honey on the 96's – or yours?

When you work in the service of your own objectives, rather than executing someone else's agenda or playing a bit part in destiny's long-running soap opera, you don't *have* to lift a finger. Only once the compulsion mechanism is disabled can genuine choice flourish.

And with choice comes freedom and accountability.

Although the 'a' word causes all of us to baulk at times, once we remove the cultural overlay of authority figures, customs and notions of honour, the fear of socially visible failure so often associated with accountability is dramatically diluted. Indeed, without the schoolroom reductionism of pass/fail, accountability (authorship, responsibility, etc) becomes an enervating motivation – an invitation to proceed.

The thing about pointlessness is that it doesn't care about success, failure, moral backbone, tremendous riches, or even beauty. There are no great rewards on offer. Neither are there any punishments pending. Understand this at the start of every project and you will invest your increasingly precious minutes and hours knowing what the real nature of the potential returns are.

When you are clear about the returns – your path towards them becomes clearer.

So, are we ready to take that gimp mask off? To start projects for joy – not just to meet the mortgage? Are you ready to inhabit the existential space formerly dominated by all those tired old meanings? Ready to write your own story of what, why and with whom?

If you answered *fuck yeah* I'd almost be tempted to honour your achievement – except that achievement is an empty cultural fetish that has no ultimate value. Instead, I'll just wish you luck.

4.
THE NARRATIVE PALLIATIVE

or

Numbed down & dumbed down: when the moral
of the story becomes a gateway drug

Therefore, just as childhood bedtime stories help kids
get to sleep for the night, their parallel adult fairy tales
help grown-ups to go to sleep forever.
Sorta like a pre-death sedative.

In this chapter I highlight the ubiquitous perils of narrative (stories) and examine our nigh universal and willing enslavement to the controlling imperatives of gods, destiny and social approval. In addition, I argue that in pure cost/benefit terms discarding common notions of meaning and purpose will help you be free and increase your probability of happiness.

The emergence of the story:

The human is a storytelling animal. Although opinion is divided as to the precise origins and initial purposes of the narrative habit, it is evident that stories also played (and continue to play) an important psycho-social function; not only as conduits and stores of information but as a way of understanding and re-framing events and experience, and crucially, as a means of reinforcing herd identity and affiliation. Combine this with our manifold fears and our capacity for both competition *and* empathy, and you have the emotional fuel required to make these yarns utterly compelling. By the time we invented representational painting (30-35 thousand years ago) we had also evolved a capacity for highly symbolic communication. In other words, an understanding that 'thing a' is a proxy for 'thing b'. Thus, stories became more than mere reportage; they symbolised broader ideas otherwise not contained in the detail of the telling. In this way, stories began to point at, or represent, uber-meanings and deeper cultural values. Through this prism, the evolution of narrative can be considered as nothing less than the invention and consolidation of tribal and personal identities – ongoing and unbroken ancestral lines that transcended the individual lifespan and, in a sense, survived the certainty of physical death. Indeed, perhaps the story is a response to adversity, a way of dealing with pain.

Those of us fortunate enough to have had loving parents who read to us at night will remember the deep thrill and calming satisfaction of a good bedtime story. In the thrall of these early stories we journeyed to perfect worlds, neatly bounded and predictable realms where events seemed to move along in a definite linear arc and there appeared to be some clear and unambiguous point or purpose to everything. In short, a world quite unlike this one. Or rather, like we wish this one would be.

As grown-ups we like to believe that our taste for these cosy confections has waned and that as the years have ticked by we have learnt to deal better with the ambiguities and ambivalence of reality – but we would be kidding ourselves. Look around and what do you see everywhere in every human culture that ever existed? Stories – and plenty of them. Linear, beginning/middle/end constructions with simple cause/effect mechanisms clustered around a central organising principle and intended to make a point. (The moral of the story and so on.) The ubiquitous practise of telling ourselves stories is central to the way in which we come to understand the world and, more directly, ourselves.

The fact that our adult stories are more complex than our infant ones only makes them more persuasive. More like reality. Like they might actually *be* real. Indeed, our addiction to the reductionist reassurance of narrative manifests itself in everything from religious and political orthodoxy to classical deterministic mathematics, from earnest self-improvement mantras to the stubborn persistence of formulaic, puerile plotlines in Hollywood movies. In fact, so hooked are we on the safety seeking, edited mechanism of narrative that we have re-exported this learned behaviour and, as a result, anthropomorphised the entire universe in the neat 'plot and point' style of a soothing bedtime yarn. By an act of grand hubristic delusion we have largely convinced ourselves that we live in a universe that parallels our own tiny experience, personalising reality according to criteria that are almost entirely subjective, highly dubious and inescapably infantile.

Now before we all hang our heads in collective philosophical shame, let's remember that our animal brains have evolved to recognise, prioritise and cross reference all manner of patterns. The brain sorts and edits data flow to give us not only an ordered sense of the world but a coherent notion of self. This is the bedrock of survivability. Without a minimum level of predictability we would have no way of orienting ourselves around the external world and no sense of persistent identity, let alone sanity. Whether you're a materialist or an idealist, it is plain that our sense of ourselves as conscious, enduring entities operating in a comprehensible world is the result of our innate ability to detect and extrapolate patterns.

In this context our virtually unquestioned acceptance of the narrative model can be understood as an evolutionary endowment, a brilliant sensory and psychological survival tool that packs together a pragmatic and powerful vision of reality that enables us to react to, plan for and successfully predict all manner of eventualities. After all, narrative is just an ordered sequence – a patterned selection of events, relationships or ideas that transfigure a messy, complex and impersonal reality into a simpler, tidier, more compact form.

The problem only really arises when narrative is conflated with meaning and self-importance, when the moral of the story migrates from bedtime to full time. When the infantile comfort bear is carried forward into adulthood and when the analgesic, sleep-inducing effect of a pretty little story becomes confused with ultimate truth and life purpose and sustains an over-inflated sense of our own significance.

However, even this proclivity wouldn't be especially dangerous were it not for the fact that the most pervasive and popular narratives all revolve around external ordination. In other words, the appeal to a higher, outside authority. As social primates we are in the nigh blind habit of bailing to the external as our go to source of personal validation, theoretical proof and super objective; as though the central legitimising force of these stories is the fact that God says, destiny decrees and society rubber stamps.

By doing this we not only give our power away but, crucially, abdicate personal responsibility. Indeed, the latter may well be considered a perverse reward for the former, for our ongoing capitulation to outside forces. We remain in a child-like state of dependence on what we might call 'the parental/external authority complex' for the reassurances of identity, predictability and meaning – although for eating our existential greens we do get to enjoy the ice cream of blaming 'others' (deities, presidents, traditions, etc) for anything and everything.

But why? What, ultimately – aside from blame shifting and righteous indignation – is the bottom line benefit? Drilling down, we eventually get back to the central denial I spoke about in previous chapters; namely, the tendency of every spiritual and secular tradition to blunt the hard edge of mortality. To pretend we don't really die. If the world is like a person, then not only are we special, almost by default, but this 'person universe' must surely have something more in mind for us than the mundane birth/death cycle inflicted upon everything else. *We* must be the exceptions.

Therefore, just as childhood bedtime stories help kids get to sleep for the night, their parallel adult fairy tales help grown-ups to go to sleep forever. Sorta like a pre-death sedative.

So, if you find yourself believing that you can't live the life you truly want because either your God, your politics, the call of duty or just the 'way of things' prevents you, it's time to jettison socially imposed 'should narratives' and write your own stories. Time to take back your power *and* its less sexy sounding companion: personal accountability.

Easier said than done, you might think. Sure, if you're a young Afghani girl growing up amidst mullah-approved violent misogyny or a civilian whose town is being bombed in the name of democracy, theocracy or ethnicity, then you do indeed have a solid real world reason not to be 'in your power', so to speak. However, let's admit it, much of what I'm discussing here reflects the exceptionally comfortable and frankly complacent perspective of the over-indulged Western middle class. That said, this is the very cohort of luxury-fattened souls who will likely comprise the principal audience for this book. (Howdy peeps.) Although most of them won't like to hear it so bluntly confessed, their lingering discontent is – like mine used to be – relatively petulant and lazy when compared to the economic, cultural and gun-wielding authoritarian travails that confront lower caste Indians, indigenous Australians and billions of others on this planet.

It is perhaps one of the ironies of Western liberal individualism that, having created (and expropriated) the wherewithal necessary to drive both the technology and social/economic conditions needed to underpin the consumer-oriented culture we now 'enjoy', we find ourselves in a state of widespread disaffection. In a zeitgeist riven with fantastical and contradictory narratives of obese self-importance and cosmic subservience.

In a very real way, most Westerners live in a permanently infantile state – at once pampered into believing they're "so fucking special" and yet almost entirely dependent on forms of parental/external authorisation to make them feel secure and give them a reason to keep working, go shopping and refrain from blowing their brains out.

This is not to say that people living in Chad or China aren't prey to the same follies – they evidently are – but let's be honest, here in the West we have far greater access to the cell door keys than most Africans or Asians currently do. Our imprisonment is largely voluntary – despite what the slavery-loving conspiracy junkies enjoy telling you.

That said, the purpose of this book isn't to mire us all in a bog of inevitable, shame-faced defeat – I'll leave that to the aforementioned conspiracists – but rather to outline a conceptual and practical path to liberation. To being an existential grown up who no longer requires apron strings and bedtime stories.

I WANNA BE ENSLAVED

Before we entirely discard our storybook, let's remind ourselves of some of the most common and dangerous narratives that keep the vast majority of us on the treadmill. Most revolve around straightforward external ordination/validation – should narratives – and some are outright slave narratives. In addition, there's the holy war/end of days story so beloved of jihadis, doomsday preppers and golden age types. All involve a degree of legislated compulsion, a dose of righteousness and a corresponding refusal to accept either mortality or responsibility.

You will note that many of these overlap or appear to counteract (or contradict?) one another. What's more, you will observe that the list below is not exhaustive – because my intention here is not to be encyclopaedic but indicative. Anyway, I'm sure you'll get the point, so without further ado here are the main chapter headings in our adult anthology of servitude and denial.

- Gods & other numinous entities – creators, angels & spirit guides insist that I do this.
- Afterlife & reincarnation – death is not the end – I am an immortal spirit, etc.
- Destiny – everything is written and happens for a reason – there are no accidents.
- Higher & life purposes – the universe has a plan for me – I'm here to do … whatever.
- Enlightenment & self-improvement – I need to evolve, man – happier, healthier, wiser, etc.
- Good & evil – light vs dark – there is a morally superior (better) way and I'm (not) choosing it.
- Attainment – gotta do, gotta go – must have, must be – gonna be #1 – get that guy – count up the likes.
- Status & power – I'm famous – don't mess with me – isn't my dick huge? – check out my bling, bitch.
- Custom – this is how it's done round here – we've always done it like this – it's clearly the best way.
- Honour & face – I must be seen to be right – be the alpha – be approved of – be with the in group.
- Wealth & trinkets – I'm rich, so fuck me – money = success = good person = happiness, etc.

As if that wasn't enough, there are some very particular and highly pessimistic slave narratives doing the rounds. Whilst they masquerade as superior and subversive insights acceptable only to a fearless elect, (oddly enough, mainly malcontent suburbanites fed on internet half-truths and shocking video 'evidence'), they are in fact defeatist tracts that allow their adherents to blame the system for just about everything and remain rooted in ironically passive alt-smugness. Whilst these 'poison world' viewpoints almost invariably contain germs of truth, their extreme ideological reading usually results in a kind of paralysing paranoia.

- Conspiracy – the 0.1% control everything – even history is a part of their cunning plan – climate change is a Chinese plot – damn those Jewish bankers (but hey, we're not Nazis) – the Queen is a lizard – all news is propaganda (except this) – oh, and everything else you've ever been told is also a lie (except this) – and if you don't believe me you're just one of the sheeple.

- Doomsday – it's all fucked – the lesbian cyborg Muslims are taking over, so let's just party till the apocalypse – maybe stock up on baked beans, batteries & bullets – God's gonna turn up in a flying pyramid and hit delete on everything soon – the Yellowstone super volcano is gonna blow – peak oil, over-population, Greenland glacial meltdown, asteroid strikes, and so it goes.

Overstated and hysterical though these kinds of narratives clearly are, the most spectacular and immediately dangerous storybook delusions are the apocalyptic fantasies of radical religion. This is the narrative of the holy warrior – be they Christian, Muslim or New Age crusaders. It posits the notion that we are living in the shadow of imminent and epochal destruction and that only a tiny cadre of specially selected jihadis will make it into the new, post 'end of everything' world. In the name of such millenarian madness all manner of violence and depravity is authorised, with eternal rewards on offer for those with enough gumption to throw gay people off buildings, feed arsenic to their children or dob their elderly relatives into the thought police.

Of course I am highlighting these extreme and ridiculous examples to underscore the driving similarities that bind both the bizarre and the more benign together. I am not for one moment suggesting that your average suburban believer in destiny is about to start decapitating their less fatalistic neighbours or stockpiling weaponry in their walk-in-robe but, rather, that the thing which our mild-mannered middle class friends have in common with their martyrdom-seeking cohorts is fear, denial and wilful delusion. (Oh, and conflation, false equivalence and gullibility.)

None of these people want to accept the universe for the gloriously impersonal, beautifully mathematical and inherently unpredictable and uncontrollable event that it is. All of them are so scared of death that they concoct an ideological perimeter fence of afterlives, self-glorifying monumentalism, vanity driven attainments and ego-serving wisdom. Indeed, everything from the shallow 'me, me, me' fetish of the West to the self-denying, rule bound 'face' culture of East Asia involves a fundamental subjugation to external authority – a master/slave relationship encapsulated in the stories we tell ourselves.

Yet, when we boil off the clutter of the finer details what we are left with are a couple of primary 'Essentialist' impulses that run through all these tales. The first is to regard the universe (existence, reality, the world, call it what you will) as a person – as having human-like conscious intentions. The second is to suppose that the universe is here *for a reason*; that there is a grand cosmic purpose that we're all a part of, and that when existence has run its course all will somehow be revealed.

Both of these are perfectly understandable habits. We are more or less bound to regard everything in relation to ourselves – in the context of humanness – and to frame everything from our science to our spiritual musings in the 'language' of the only experience we know.

Quite clearly this is a limited perspective, a small and very idiosyncratic window on the vast panoply of existence – and given the obviously oceanic hugeness of everything it is little wonder we have reacted to our own miniscule and tenuous place in the scheme of things by overlaying a very human patina of meaning. The purpose of this interpretive smear is more about making ourselves feel important in the face of the infinitude than it is about explaining the hidden subtext of the cosmos. In turn, the 'delusion of mattering' helps us to stave off the brutal egalitarian certainty of death and of the fact that our lives are just events. Shit that's happening.

Some of you will doubtless recall how in the last chapter I spoke about the idea of pointlessness being a key to freedom. For most of us that seems counter-intuitive. As action-oriented animals purposeless idling strikes us as boring at best, suicidally nihilistic at worst, and rarely, if ever, fulfilling. This book is here to help free you from that idea.

Because meaning is slavery and self-importance is a masochistic self-punishment device.

In this regard, the palliative of narrative has the side effect of dependence. Whilst the opiate of a good yarn – with its self-contained prescription for the existential blues – helps us to dull the pain and stress associated with mortality, uncertainty and insignificance, and gives us an important role to play in the unfolding of an essentially meaningful cosmic drama, it also traps us in the errant child role; always somehow falling short of expectation and drifting off-purpose.

It's like this: Because it's all supposed to be about something I'm constantly in danger of getting it wrong – of missing the point. And because I matter, it matters whether or not I fuck it up. The universal parent, it seems, will never be truly satisfied. I will always be a slave to its whims; constantly in danger of failing the existential exam.

THE CULT OF COSMIC PERSONALITY

We all see how readily children personalise their world – naming their toys, humanising the household pets and so on – but we might not recognise that as adults we have refined and extended this reflex. Perhaps we no longer have invisible friends or speak to the stuffed bear as though it was a living thing but we are still in the habit of anthropomorphising everything from animal behaviour to cosmic history. It is this process of imbuing the external with human ego – with I – that creates and sustains gods and underpins the narratives of destiny and higher purpose.

Since the 'I' is the most immediate and, perhaps, the only thing we have, it is not surprising that we extend it back out into the external world from which we first learnt about it. For just as we discover our sense of who we are via the mechanism of our initial engagements with the wider world – or the Not I – so we later colonise the universe by configuring it in terms that reflect the parameters and objectives of the I. Unsurprisingly, the colour and feel of our relationship with this vast externalised I mirrors that of the foundational infant relationships we share with our parents, siblings and significant others. In other words, without fully realising it, we set up a mode of self-regarding that mimics the values, judgements and language of those important others, and by extension, we overlay this learned internal schema back out onto the external. No wonder God so often resembles a fuming parent and that the plan the universe has for us is so linear and pedagogic. It's as though existence were a kind of kindergarten and destiny a series of pre-planned play activities, with the child care workers as God's police, always ready to use 'wait till I tell your parents' as a threat of punishing Heavenly retribution.

Feeling like a naughty girl now? Like a bad little boy?

What astounds me most about this almost Freudian architecture is not so much its existence, or even its prevalence, but that it's so consistently didactic, disciplinarian and defeatist. Sure, the notion of 'world as person' has the benefit of making things seem comprehensible and the universe not so coldly indifferent, but unfortunately the coin of personalisation is double sided – and for every death defying, philosophical sidestep we invent there's a basket of other human traits that come along with it; namely, judgement, lies, denial and control.

Let's ponder that toxic quartet a moment – the better to see them for what they are. Judgement, lies and denial are all means of control. We've all met people who use these weapons and we all understand that they are generally employed to shore up the user's position. We may even use them ourselves – although perhaps without realising. However, many of us still struggle to see (let alone accept) that culturally and individually we have programmed these same characteristics into the source code of meaning and morality, thereby creating a rod of ritual punishment for ourselves. Judging ourselves according to externally imposed measures. Lying to ourselves about how excruciatingly precious we are – and how everything we do is so very important. Denying our mortal animality to the point of hubris and using the fantasy of control in a futile attempt to whitewash ambiguities and reduce uncertainties to a set of neat narrative panaceas.

Yet what a price we pay for our pain relieving concoctions; for the cute little bedtime universe we like to be tucked up in.

- The ever-present oversight of the other – God, the universe, big daddy, the Illuminati, my friends, work colleagues, my partner, even my kids are watching me – comparing me – judging me – making sure I don't let them down or show them up – reminding me where I'm going wrong – obliging me – guilt tripping me – punishing me.

When we personalise the other – creating the great parental/external I – we set up an amorphous, all-seeing authority complex which then proceeds to drone on relentlessly at us for not being enough this or being too much that. It clearly has an objective in mind for us (if only we weren't too stupid or selfish to notice) and has legislated a selection of readily available, socially visible roles for us to fulfil while we endeavour to pass their arcane cosmic examination.

What's more, if we buy into their afterlife story – call it Heaven, Hell or transmigration – we condemn ourselves to an *eternity* of being a repeated disappointment to this magnificent existential parent figure.

Okay, so they pat us on the head with a 'there, there, you're not gonna die' and a 'you're so important to me' but boy do they extract a price for the spiritual paracetamol they serve up.

Hey, I'm gonna crush this pill up and spoon it to you with strawberry jam, so you better fucking pull your socks up and get about realising your divine mission, you unworthy little fuck – or I'm gonna make you do it again and again until you get it right. Or maybe I'll just shove white hot pitchforks up your arse for the rest of forever. Your choice, mofo!

If that sounds a little overcooked, check out Yahweh. No disrespect to my Jewish and Israeli friends but a scan of the Old Testament reveals a litany of genocidal, racist, sexist, homophobic, slave-owning, incestuous, autocratic brutality better befitting the psychopaths of pulp fiction than a benevolent heavenly father. Ask yourself what possessed us to posit such a wantonly vicious creator to oversee our every activity, inner and outer?

I mean, a gentle maternal goddess ready with the opiates to soothe our mortal dread and make us feel as though we mean something, sure – but an unhinged, vengeful bully who regularly seeks recourse to (and condones) murder, rape, enslavement and mass drowning? WTF?

Again, before you dismiss this as an extreme example, let's remember that Yahweh (Jehovah) features hugely in all three Abrahamic faiths – Judaism, Christianity and Islam – and is therefore deep in the cultural and psychological background of something like 3.8 billion people (or just a shade under half the total population).

What does this tell us? Taking the existence of Yahweh and all other 'personal' numina out of the equation, this leaves us with ourselves. With *our* desire for control and order, for certainty and clearly delineated roles, for mandated purpose and the ultimate, external tick of approval.

Drill down a little further and you come across a deep and nagging seam, a bedrock need for love and acceptance – to be in the in group. Just what you'd expect from a bunch of social mammals.

And what does the herd confer upon the individual? In evolutionary terms: protection, mating opportunities and shared knowledge. In more nuanced and conscious social terms: belonging. For each there is a price. As there is for everything.

THE FASCISM OF MEANING

You will no doubt be familiar with the hackneyed, disposable saying 'everything happens for a reason' or its equally inane sibling 'there are no accidents'. Although there *are* still credible, well-structured and entirely deterministic models being debated in the theoretical physics community, you can be sure that the people who spout these so-called wisdoms are thinking more spiritually than scientifically. Their contention is not mathematic, neither Quantum nor Newtonian, nor even as rudimentary as cause and effect. Rather, what they are saying is that everything is unfolding *as it should*. According to a plan. For a reason, or set of reasons, pre-determined at some point by an agency with remarkably human proclivities and agendas. (This is sometimes called Essentialism.)

The hilarious irony in all this off-the-rack spiritualism is that the people who repeat it and Tweet it as though it were a kind of countercultural statement of dizzying insight are in fact arguing for exactly the kind of rigorous, cosmological determinism that their apparently evolved consciousness pretends to abhor. To make matters worse, their beloved existential slavery is imbued with a moral tone. For these poor dumb robots of karma the whole universe sits in judgement of them, so that not only are their sins supposedly inevitable (they happen for a reason, right?) but also, somewhat viciously, punishable. Ouch!

It bewilders me why anybody bothers to sign up to such an avowedly bad deal. Well actually, it doesn't really. You see, what the glove puppets of destiny are really looking for is meaning.

What's wrong with that? you ask. Surely we can forgive folk for wanting to suffuse their lives with a sense of meaning? Better that than just treading water until an otherwise pointless existence comes to an end and it all turns out to have been for nothing. Absolutely yes. And no at the same time.

Whilst the idea of meaning is incredibly useful on a psycho-emotional level as both a motivator and existential painkiller, the architecture of meaning is such that it typically necessitates an external validating force to be, yep, meaningful. In its most common form life meaning or super objective is understood as either the execution of an historical strategy (God's plan, what I'm here for, it's meant to be, etc), or as a vainglorious desire for legacy (fame, making the kids proud, being remembered, etc). In Eastern religions and their New Age copies this can also be translated as the working off of karmic debts; reducing life to a moral repayment plan. In other words, life as a form of punishment for earlier transgressions. A refresher course for poorly performing souls.

Thus, the most popular and virulent manifestations of meaning are all social – by which I mean they all exist solely in the context of external and visible measures, as opposed to being purely private inventions without recourse to gods, divine plans, peer approval or socially defined notions of success, morality or status.

Boiling it down further, we arrive at the vague but pervasive sense that life must surely be *about* something. There must be an *outcome*. As though it were a story. A sweet little bedtime story, no less – with its neat, contrived conclusions all tied to some basic moral. Where unambiguous binaries like good and evil, or on purpose and missing the point, make muddy waters seem crystal clear.

Of course, this 'aboutness' is entirely anthropocentric – with meaning based on *human* experience. On *human* frailty. As a means of centralising the haphazard, episodic mess of living onto a plotline – into a coherent narrative.

As such, meaning is a mode of control; and, since virtually all of us derive our sense of meaning and purpose from the external, the locus of that control is also external.

However, even if we do derive our overarching sense of life purpose from entirely personal criteria, we are saddled with the proverbial cross to bear. To have clearly defined, short-dated projects which don't quite work out is one thing – a disappointment perhaps, a lesson maybe – but to fall short in the pursuit of life's ultimate point? Fuuuuck, *that's* heavy.

In this frame it's easy to see how meaning works neatly with the background radiation of punishing deities, admonishing parents, bucket list must mania, enlightenment snobbery and the ubiquity of mortal dread. Indeed, it turns out that the fantasy of meaning is a fascist meta-narrative.

And why fascist? Consider the Latin root of the word; *fasces* means bundle and is usually represented visually by a cluster of wooden rods bundled together with an axe. In ancient Rome this symbolised the power of a magistrate and was associated with jurisdiction. In other words: external, socially mandated judgement backed by enforcement. No surprise that for the last century fascism has been inextricably linked with brutal totalitarianism. Need I say more?

As for the 'meta' part, consider what all the narratives we've been discussing in this chapter are underpinned by. Whatever else they're trying to say, they are united in suggesting that their particular prescription is for a life of *meaning*. For a *universe* of meaning. Whether it's shop till you drop, being top dog or fulfilling your divine higher purpose, the background narrative is that meaning is generated and sustained outside of us. That it is innate. Essential. That it is a form of imperative. That it is the very *point* of things. The why.

So, my advice is to overthrow the fascist yoke of meaning and embrace futility and pointlessness. Allied with a fear free attitude to death this will liberate you from the morphine of narrative and, as a consequence, give you the psychological muscle required to ignore convention, subvert socially ordained roles, stop playing stupid status games and get over the dictatorship of should. Or, to put it more upliftingly, to live how you damn well choose.

MEANING & NARRATIVE THROUGH A RISK / REWARD PRISM

Given that this book seeks to bring economic clarity to the otherwise misty realms of spirituality, it is only right that we turn our focus now to the risk metrics of the narrative palliative.

Whilst the PHI – Potential Happiness Index – we outlined in Chapter 2 is adequate for clarifying the relative values we place upon things like ambition, obligation and relationships it doesn't directly address the cost/benefit of continuing to wed yourself to the meaning and narrative school.

Here again, as with the PHI, I delegate the ascribing of all relative value weightings to you because regardless of what I may or may not believe, it's your life, your happiness, etc. Instead, I shall simply list the pluses and minuses of swallowing the narrative pill and buying into the meaning mantra.

In addition, for the sake of brevity, I have deemed meaning and narrative to be equivalent for the purposes of this exercise – because, as we have already established, meaning *is* a kind of external ordination narrative.

However, before we get listing, I can declare that my base level assumptions here are that there is no personal god and that the universe and all of us are not here for a reason. Gods and reasons are invented by humans for entirely human ends. Furthermore, I do not believe in destiny or its judgemental moralising equivalent – karma – and hold that death is quite simply death; namely, the end. Oblivion. That said, the cost/benefit split on page 64 remains a useful analytic lens, regardless of your particular set of beliefs.

The benefits of narrative:

- Lessens the pain and fear associated with death.
- Creates an externally validating framework – sometimes approves of you & your choices.
- Creates an externally guiding framework – creates structure & gives clear direction.
- Makes you feel important.
- 'Warms' up the universe – the universe takes an interest in you – is imbued with personality.
- Allows you to avoid responsibility – cos it's all part of a plan – blame it on the system.
- Deals neatly with uncertainties – defuses the fear of the unknown.
- Deals with the nagging sense of futility – it all means something.
- Helps you to feel right about stuff – wise, enlightened, etc.
- Helps you to fit in – cos virtually everyone else believes this shit – plays this game.
- Promises you eternal life – no death.

The costs of narrative:

- Sets up a punishing parental/external authority complex – always telling you off.
- Sets you up to fail – because you'll never really be good enough.
- Weds your self-esteem to externally approved outcomes.
- Weighs you down with 'should' – obliges you to stick with the programme – enslaves you.
- Keeps you in an infantile state of dependence & fear – incessant approval seeking.
- Makes you prone to ideological excess, cruelty & intolerance.
- Makes you vulnerable to conspiratorial paranoia – and associated defeatist whinging.
- Pushes you to conform to societal norms.
- Keeps you on the treadmill.
- Engages you in endless status games – professionally, personally, socially, etc.
- Diverts you into the pursuit of stuff that won't make you happy – trinkets, status, etc.
- Weds you to a massive edifice of denial – the puncturing of which can be catastrophic.
- Gives predators the cover they need to keep abusing you – tradition, shame, etc.
- Threatens eternal damnation – you'll fucking wish you were dead.

Therefore, if you, like so many of us in the West, feel that you're just not living the life you would truly like to, or that you are postponing potential happiness until *after* you've paid the mortgage, lost the weight or got the promotion, ask yourself about the value of the narratives you adhere to. Are they worth the cost you pay in slavish obedience, self-punishment and the sheer energy involved in maintaining a buffer zone of denial? Does the fantasy of meaning adequately compensate you for subjugating yourself to the lecturing, linear command and control voices of external authority? Is the existence of the bucket list worth the gut twisting envy, crushing loss of esteem and sense of lifetime disappointment that almost always accompanies the must imperative?

And so it goes. We can frame the question in a number of ways but it will always centre on the notion of value. Of risk versus reward.

Think of your belief system (world view, narrative library, etc) as a bet – a psycho-emotional investment portfolio designed to make life more pleasant and reduce the shock of setbacks and unforeseens. Whatever else they are, our beliefs – yours and mine alike – are a coping mechanism. A survival tool. A compass. A pain killer. However strongly or mildly we hold them, we are not only wagering that our beliefs are more likely to be true than false but also betting that sticking to them will deliver the goods in terms of happiness, (sense of meaning, feeling good about ourselves, courage to pursue what we really love, etc).

In saying this I am specifically excluding things like the 'belief' in gravity (if I hurl myself from the cliff top I will accelerate at 9.8m/s/s towards the centre of the Earth), and other stuff that we can safely regard as facts … but *in*clude the clearly self-defeating and miserablist beliefs of conspiracy slaves, poor me types and apocalypse lovers. Even though these belief systems are clearly doomful, disempowering and even dangerous there is a psychological pay-off for the believer. They have emotionally invested in their hopeless situation and/or righteous rage and most likely have neatly formed narratives that support this strategy. For them, the perceived rewards of being a victim outweigh what we might consider to be the all too obvious costs.

Either way, the point here isn't about the rightness or wrongness of certain beliefs. Indeed, since notions of right and wrong are invariably wedded to our self-serving biases – not to mention severely limited by the Lilliputian window we all have on reality – we are free to assess risk/reward questions in terms that have an impact upon us and our happiness without fretting too much about whether there really *is* a god or if vaccines are indeed a plot to make your kids autistic.

Okay, so for the record, here's the narrative rethink that helped me to negate the fear of death, escape the prison of meaning, walk away from delusional self-importance and free myself from the socially imposed 'need' to achieve, compete and own stuff – the upshot of which has been a life-altering sense of freedom and a greatly increased potential for enriching experience and happiness.

At its core, this shift involved an *emotional* acceptance of a suite of related realisations that, although intellectually easy to comprehend, had previously proved psychologically impossible to integrate. It began, of course, with a full and ultimately grateful acceptance of mortality. With the notion that my inevitable death – my ephemerality – is what gives my life its value. Its oomph. That my death will also be a kind of release. A simple end. A return to the great nothing. The ultimate liberation.

Once I had honestly and fully accepted the certainty of my own demise – without recourse to afterlives, reincarnations or enlightenment sophistry to blunt the finality – it became apparent that my erstwhile addiction to the ideologies of grandiose purpose (meaning) and spiritual uplift (wisdom) was the baseline driver behind the raft of self-imprisoning narratives that were fuelling my sense of dread, failure, impatience, incompleteness, worthlessness and obligation.

In addition, it soon became clear to me that by embracing mortality with gratitude I could release myself from the burden of self-importance. From the ordeal of mattering and the reductive dictatorship of meaning. In fact, from all external ordination narratives. From the desire to please and appease the pantheon of social/cosmic authority figures. And then, look what else soon got dropped:

- The desire to be the best – compete, achieve, out do, out think, be cool, etc.
- The desire for approval – recognition, acclamation, admiration, etc.
- The desire to be right – wise, enlightened – be the saviour, great leader, etc.
- The desire for higher purpose & life meaning.
- The idea that anything is intrinsically important.
- The passive acceptance of socially received imperatives.

Ecstatic Nihilism

If asked to label it, I'd say that my current 'philosophy' is Ecstatic Nihilism. What this means is that my response to the idea that life is an essentially meaningless phenomenon has been a frequently euphoric sense of lightness and liberation. Minus the pre-ordained meaning objective I am free to pursue 'for the sake of it' activities and, more importantly, to empower an authentic self-narrative. For me, pointlessness and futility make room for genuinely honest values to arise. True, this is also a narrative; a meta-narrative that dispenses with the usual linear reductions of morality, functionality or dénouement – and significantly, mutes all judgement and should mantras.

NB: To dig a little deeper into this – and into what I call 'the ecstasy of nothingness' – see Appendix 3.

In pure risk/reward terms this struck me as a big win because, even though I could not be *100% certain* that I'm not here for a reason, by changing my existential investment strategy from a narrative/meaning based portfolio to a 'nothing matters, everything is ultimately pointless' position I effectively granted myself carte blanche to live life more or less exactly as I wished to.

Viewed through the lens of emotion, this shift removed (or at least dramatically reduced) the impact of fear.

Lose the horror of death and the fear of disapproval, failure or getting it wrong and suddenly a huge weight is lifted. Should narratives no longer have any coercive power.

Now you may well be thinking that all I've done is change narratives – and you would be right. Mine is now the narrative of what I have loosely come to call Ecstatic Nihilism and guess what … just like immortality promising gods my embrace of pointlessness reconciles me with the fact that I will one day die. Ta-dah!

The key difference however, isn't in the afterlife or the realm of spiritual truth but in the here and now. In the lounge room. In the queue at the supermarket. On Monday mornings. Right now, typing out this sentence, writing this book because it fits in with my story about myself. Just because I well want to.

So ask yourself this:

- Do my narratives shackle me to external authorisation and to sources of validation and meaning, or, do they allow me to live the life I truly desire and be the person I really want to be?

And:

- Are my narrative choices principally underpinned by my various fears, doubts and craving for acceptance and approval?

Having answered these questions in the privacy of your own reflection ask yourself again if the bet you've made on the rightness of these stories is worth the price you pay in time, effort and sense of wellbeing?

Remember, narratives, beliefs and purposes can be changed. They are just stories, after all. So if your narrative palliative isn't serving you well and the side effects are too severe, flush the pills down the toilet. And if that bedtime story is giving you nightmares, ask Mummy and Daddy to read you another one.

NOTE TO SELF:

The *possibility* of being wrong is not worth the *experience* of living a shit life.

5.
TIME FOR LIVING

or

Your impending death has set you free
(now you just need to accept it)

Suppose the looming certainty of your death
gave you the ultimate imprimatur:
a licence to live without fear.

In this chapter I endeavour to diffuse the fear of death by revealing not only how futile it is but how mortal dread ties us to externalised authority and its socially or divinely mandated objectives. When we run the risk metrics over mortal terror, it becomes clear that adopting a grateful attitude to your upcoming death allows you to truly and fully live.

So why *do* we invest so much of our time into the ongoing promulgation and justification of the external authorisation complex, that edifice of custom, socially visible attainment and Essentialist imperative that keeps so many of us in a child-like state of approval seeking?

True, our social and gendered animality hardwires a compulsion to belong – and indeed plays a pivotal role in forming our very notion of identity – but surely, as adults, once we consciously acknowledge and understand these evolutionary drivers, we should no longer be such obvious suckers for the parental/external and its endless should narratives.

Of course there is no single and simple answer to this. The ubiquity of what is sometimes called Essentialism – namely, the idea that truths, meanings, purposes, etc, are woven into the very fabric of existence – reflects a number of psycho-emotional pre-dispositions. Amongst them:

- Lots of people like being slaves – they get to abdicate personal responsibility – blame the system – use the 'God made me' excuse – cop out by insisting it was 'written', etc.
- Lots of people don't trust their own judgement – they need an external source of agreement and validation – a tick from the teacher – a Godly gold star – please tell me I'm right, etc.
- Most of us hate the idea of being alone – fear of exile/exclusion – conformity = approval / approval = happiness – being different gets you disliked – makes you a target, etc.

    +

- Personalising the universe makes the world seem less scary – if everything can be understood as a kind of 'person' (with likes/dislikes, plans and so on) it won't seem so unknowable – so dangerous.
- Destiny enshrines a sense of greater purpose – I am part of a great, unfolding story – there is a role for me – therefore I matter, etc.

In my view though, what lurks deep in the weave of all this is our old bete noir – death. The parental/external architecture outlined above (and in previous chapters) exists in synergy with the central denial; that proclivity we have for finding ways to either pretend we don't or ignore that we *will* die. Indeed, our desperate and absurd desire not to die is a key ingredient in our almost universal

69

investment in externalised higher authority mechanisms. This has driven us to invent all manner of religions, philosophies and wishful 'science'; anything that might preserve us.

Here again I am not seeking to denigrate or pathologise the desire to persist. Indeed, humans are not alone in this. Nor indeed are organisms. For just as homeostasis refers to organic systems that seek to maintain a nearly constant state of internal balance, so too complex atomic structures (compounds) generally 'seek' to maintain their form. The forces governing electro-chemical and electro-magnetic interactions have thrown up countless gazillions of formations that effectively resist the underlining entropic trend. Everything from rocks to planets to stars provides us with evidence of identifiably persisting structures in a permanently changing universe. Though our best current models tend to suggest that entropy will eventually win out, it is abundantly clear that things 'like' to stay principally as they are for as long as they can. (Indeed, we see this reflected in Newton's first law of motion, or law of inertia. *An object at rest stays at rest and an object in motion stays in motion with the same speed and direction unless acted upon by an unbalanced force.*)

What's more, if we permit ourselves wriggle room for metaphysical musing, we can envisage all of existence as a dynamic disequilibrium; the result of an interaction between the fundamental forces of persistence and change – the tension between the oppositional and seemingly polar cosmic trends of complexification and entropy. The universe, or 'existence complex', contains a whole bunch of stuff ordered so as to *be* calcium, fish, comets and so on, as well as the inexorable erosion and alteration of that order observed across time. Or, to put it more elegantly, existence is the process of Being and Time executing a sublime dance of becoming and unbecoming.

Without drifting too far into philosophical arcanery or the minutiae of physics, the upshot for us is that to be is to eventually not be. Whilst none of us have any trouble applying this to the collection of water and minerals that make up our physical bodies, we reflexively cringe from the thought that this also applies to the persistent linear narrative we call 'I'.

At their psycho-emotional core every après-vie and reincarnation story and most of the *we're all portals of the one consciousness* explanations I've ever encountered are really just

---

Self as life

Boiled down – stripped of moral and/or purpose narratives and sifted out from the obvious drama and emotion we understandably attach to it – the experience (event) we know as 'life' is indistinguishable from the experience we know as I, as the self. Our ongoing and consistent sense of self is foundationally underpinned by memory (access to saved data) and our related capacity to predict future outcomes based on the patterns revealed in that data. This holds for both the conscious and unconscious aspects of our life and identity. In a very real sense, *self is the act of mining memory to best respond to present conditions and predicted futures*. Yet, self is also the act of recognising self – I delineating itself from the Not I – and in this regard the self-awareness phenomenon we call life is predicated on our ability to receive and interpret external information; in our case, sense data. Thus, once the antennae, storage systems and retrieval mechanisms cease to function, the 'homeostatic self event system' (life) collapses. Crucially, because our highly detailed identity – our narrative of self – is also a pattern in the data flow, once that information becomes inaccessible our present, linear self event ends. Dunno about you, but I'd call that death.

thinly disguised rescue missions for the ego. Even if we *are* part of a unified super-consciousness (for instance, the universe wanting to know itself), when our present incarnation dies that's it for Darren, Sonia, Xiaoye, Mustafa or whatever you currently call yourself. The specific, encapsulated consciousness event that is *your life now* will come to its end. The homeostatic mechanisms will cease to be effective. Your existential reserve account will be spent – never to be replenished. For the present you, time itself will stop – and even if you believe that linear time is an illusion*, the illusion will also stop.

(***Re:** Time being an illusion. Do not illusions also happen in time?)

However, far from wanting to drive nails into your coffin or rub your nose into the notion of your own extinction, my goal here is replace fear and denial with gratitude and liberation. Because it's our mortal dread that keeps enslaving narratives ticking along, that keeps us on the treadmill of deluded self-importance and essential over-arching purpose. It's our existential dark matter. But it doesn't have to be that way.

Imagine if you did *not* feel at all compelled to spend your time fulfilling socially ordained objectives or playing externally defined roles in a drama of someone else's devising. Suppose the looming certainty of your death gave you the ultimate imprimatur: a licence to live without fear.

As I argued in Chapter 1, we can begin this process of liberation by realigning our notions of value, moving them from the pursuit of objects, status and so-called enlightenment to the simple currency of time. If we recognise that the most valuable commodity we have at our disposal is the dwindling supply of our days then, if we're honest, this forces a re-calibration. One corollary of this value switch, of this altered existential investment strategy, is the disempowerment of the great parental/external complex. After all, why invest your ever decreasing temporal slush fund in satisfying the infantile marketing objectives of the 'vanity and fear based' machinery of control? I mean, seriously … wtf!

From here, and as indicated in Chapter 2, we can begin a process of re-examining and disentangling the relative values we place upon some of the most salient realities affecting our lives (relationships, ethics, health, wherewithal, etc). Furthermore, by utilising the 'mathematical' formula I outlined – the Potential Happiness Index – we can begin a more pragmatic and meaningful reappraisal of the ways in which these competing values might affect our likelihood of being happy as we go forward.

In a sense, these things operate at a merely intellectual level; and like awareness without action they could easily pass by as yet another episode of more or less agreeable noise. The fire inside, the real change agent, revolves around our attitude to mortality. And I don't just mean *accepting* death in some cool, abstract fashion but profoundly *embracing* it as the wellspring of your deliverance.

All human cultures have nominated and reviled death as their number one thing to be utterly afraid of. Lies, punishment and denial have all flourished in its deadly shadow. Yet suppose we were to turn and look directly at what we are most scared of. Imagine if we were to gaze directly into the face of oblivion. And smile.

Effectively, what I'm suggesting here is a nigh heretical trinity of liberating attitudes – an all-conquering triumvirate that has, I'll be frank, handed me back my life. Or rather, imbued me with the courage to wrench it decisively away from the colonial clutches of Gods, customs, career paths and simplistic storybook narratives.

- Exalt the advent of your death – it will save you from fear.
- Embrace your utter insignificance – it will free you from chains.
- Revel in the futility & pointlessness of your existence – for now you are free to create.

Wahhabism, Salafism and why it's alright to murder innocent bystanders

Wahhabism and Salafism are both reformist schools in Sunni Islam and are variously literalist, anti-modern, anti-Shi'a and anti-European. The former was founded in the 1700s, the latter in the 1800s, and both are minority sects within the broader church of Islam. The jihadist/terrorist spectacle we have witnessed in the early part of this century has largely been driven by adherents to these hardline denominations. Like Nazis, Stalinists and honour killers everywhere, these folks are highly principled and have well-developed narratives around custom, morality, fighting supposedly evil enemies and bringing about epochal change and ideal societies. Indeed, so enamoured are they of their treasured Essentialist values, so anchored to the externally mandating authorities that green-light their actions, that they grant themselves licence to murder, rape and enslave. By subjugating themselves to the will of the higher authority (god, ism, etc), they can effectively evade personal responsibility for their cruelty; and this in turn underscores the de-humanisation of both self and victim required to make such pre-planned barbarism possible.

Of course, many would decry this as blatantly Nihilist – and I would agree. However, whereas Nihilism and its cousin Existentialism are popularly understood to be depressing and defeatist, in my experience they are profoundly liberating and optimistic prisms through which to contemplate reality and our little part in it.

Optimistic? I hear you ask. Well yeah – if you believe that assuming sole authorship and responsibility for the story of your own life, free from the dictats of numina, karma and 'must' lists, represents a better option than being a resentful, hemmed in suburbanite slave frittering your life away in a societal Skinner Box of iThings, corporate ladders and mortgage repayments – it most certainly is.

The other common criticism is that by ridding ourselves of Essentialist meaning tropes – abandoning Gods and other organs of externalised, morally engaged authority – we will automatically be thrown into an abyss that is amoral at best; or wanton, cruel and debauched at worst.

Okay, so let's kill that one off right now – and I mean *kill*.

- The Khmer Rouge's Year Zero mania of the late 1970s.
- The 100 day Hutu v Tutsi Rwandan slaughterfest of 1994.
- The Srebrenica Muslim men & boy massacre of 1995.
- The multiple murderous activities of Wahhabist/Salafist lunatics in this century alone.

Yes, that's right – just four non-Nazi examples of historically recent episodes of wanton homicidal barbarism committed by people *informed and inspired* by cherished and righteous narratives involving Gods, ethnicity and social good (that took me all of five seconds to think of). You get the point, surely? Humanity doesn't resort to cruelty when it fails to uphold tradition and respect long revered authority figures; in fact it often resorts to the most vicious of its various cruelties *because* of tradition and so-called moral imperative. Let's face it, the charnel house of human history is piled sky high with the blood-caked evidence of our numerous ideological justifications for murder, rape, imprisonment, torture ... dot, dot, dot – need I say more?

CHOOSE LIFE

Time for another potential heresy – though really this is a staggeringly banal statement of the obvious:

- Excluding those of us who are currently physically restrained, being force fed or lying in a coma, we are all absolutely 100% free – because none of us *have* to stay alive. However awful things are we can always end it. Staying alive *is* a choice.

Sure, that's an extreme and possibly outrageous thing to assert, even if it is undeniably true; but my aim here is not necessarily to convince you to commit suicide (although it's perfectly fine with me if you do) or indeed to propose some kind of death worshipping cult of romantic darkness. Rather, my intention is to help you bury the 'have to' lie. You don't *have* to do *any*thing. Ever. Death gives all us the ultimate get out key.

(Stay with me, folks – this *is* going somewhere.)

I say this because, if we're honest, hardly any of us actively *choose* life. We're here because we were born and we just cling on because we simply cannot imagine or bear the idea of not being here. We're only alive because we believe it's preferable to death. That, and the fact that our genetic construction impels us towards self-preservation at almost any cost. After all, what are pain and fear but the most strident of survival alarms. In other words, we rarely, if ever, consciously and calmly *decide* to stay alive. Mostly, living is just an unquestioned habit underwritten by a deep seam of dread.

You can hear this reflected in some of our most common sayings:

- At least I'm alive.
- Well y'know, you're a long time dead.
- While there's life, there's hope.

None of which are exactly a resounding endorsement or recognition of the extraordinarily unlikely and truly awesome phenomenon of self-aware consciousness we know as *our lives*. In fact, it's probably not too great a stretch to suggest that the fear of death sits at the primal core of our motivation – especially since, at *our* level of consciousness, we are acutely self-regarding creatures who understand at a relatively early age that we will die. True, there's also the 'go forth and multiply' imperative but really that's just the survival (persistence) instinct transposed from the specific, encapsulated I (you) to a greater self (your descendants). In essence this is us confronting death over the long term, via the agency of our species as it moves through generations – our genes imperfectly replicating themselves in an ongoing process of iterative flux.

No wonder we have created cultures and societies based on fear. For all of our rational muscle and technological ingenuity, the list of stuff that scares us remains almost endless: terrorism, crime, superbugs, immigrants, this apocalypse, that cataclysm, and so on and so on.

Yet, if we could flick a switch and come to regard death as a supreme liberation – the very certainty that instils our ephemeral existence with its fragile and extraordinary beauty – we might begin to dissolve our fear and, in that fearless state, truly and deliberately *live*, as opposed to just clinging on desperately in a futile and terrified attempt to prevent oblivion.

You may well say that this is simply a sidestep, a neat sophistry that really changes nothing or, worse, some eye-rollingly awful piece of New Age inspiro-porn. Of course, at one level it is – the level of mere words, of memes and affirmations, of comfortably middle class writers giving you the benefit of their supposed fucking insight.

Except that it's also true. Shedding our death fear and the corollary need for afterlife stories would allow us to easily dispose of all those parental/external authority figures who promise us eternal life in return for obedience and, by extension, seriously diffuse the coercive power of should in all its more Earthly manifestations.

From personal experience I can report that the removing (or at the very least, the drastic reduction) of mortal terror has triggered a similar shedding of the baggage around expectation, the search for ultimate meaning, the pressures of striving and the delusions of self-importance. As soon as I embraced the notion of my impending death with genuine gratitude, it was as though my life was handed back to me. Now, within the constraints of physics and finance and informed by a few basic ideas about being nice to people, I pretty much do whatever I want.

Again – good on paper but …

Okay, assuming that I'm not either lying or utterly deluded, how did I manage to crack this nut? Here I come back to the other two items in our aforementioned attitudinal trilogy.

Firstly, by abandoning the idea that I was somehow significant, or that God or the universe had specially endowed me with qualities that made the event of my life that much more remarkable or noteworthy than yours, I freed myself from any kind of externally imposed 'must' agenda. The pressure evaporated. I didn't especially matter in the grand scheme, so there was no need to bother with moral exams or cosmic KPIs and no onus of responsibility to history or posterity to do, be or discover anything. That left me kinda free really.

From there, it wasn't a big jump to accept that my life wasn't *about* anything. There wasn't an essentially mandated meaning of life for me to discern. The universe hadn't sent me here *for a reason* or to walk a particular, pre-ordained path; so that left me entirely at liberty to wander where I wanted for whatever reason I felt appropriate or interesting. Or even, just to dawdle aimlessly while pleasantly enjoying the view.

Put it like this: you've most likely heard the saying 'dance like nobody is watching' – all I'm doing now is living like no one's watching. Or rather, the fact that nothing matters means I'm free to choose anything.

You may think it sounds glib to say that nothing matters but remember, even if you are an Essentialist who believes there *is* an externally ordained alpha-purpose or goal, you still put your focus where *you* think it's important. Her rejection of you only hurts because her acceptance matters. That little insult only bothers you because you decided it matters what that guy thinks of you or your opinion. You're only working those long hours (in the job or on the project) because of some end goal or perceived reward that *matters* to you. What's more, given that none of us can seriously claim to know, or to have a reasonable expectation of somehow divining the *actual* truth of everything, we must, if we're honest, humbly accept that our attraction to grand meanings and super objectives is because the belief scheme associated with it somehow *matters* to us. Rewards us. (Just as my 'nothing matters' alternative does for me, if only because it enables me to be happier, calmer and more open to the simple beauty of things.)

Once we accept that all 'mattering' is simply the result of personal choosing then we can make our choices freed from the burden (or the convenient blame shifting excuse) of externally imposed importance or the pressure of being right or wrong.

Thus, returning to our old friend death, although we can now freely admit that we don't and *can't* really know what happens to us after we die, we can still say with a very high degree of certainty that the incarnated, atomised ego complex that comprises the current self-identifying consciousness event that we recognise as being life will cease when our brains stop processing sense data and allowing access to the memories that make up our not only our store of knowledge, but our very sense of a persistent and consistent I. Sure, the soul or the spirit or whatever may indeed continue in some way and in some realm, in a kind of superposition perhaps – but *not* as the currently collapsed waveform of you.

And if even *that* doesn't matter to you – bingo – freedom.

Furthermore, the death event is then transformed from a shattering finality to be dreaded and resisted with every straining fibre into an enervating invitation to enjoy with absolute liberty the beguiling, beautiful and fascinating experience of selfhood and all the sensory, emotional and intellectual glories of the external world; and all *just because*. Not ticking items off karma's list of ethical assignments to be endlessly re-submitted, or pulling your hair out trying to boil the whole universe down to a pithy catchphrase. Not conquering the corporate ladder, nor sexily improving yourself by visiting the 1001 ancient piles of rock someone insisted you photograph before you die. Just living. For the pure sake of it.

And knowing it will end and that it will all amount to nothing – and that right and wrong are, in the final analysis, irrelevant categories – renders every socially imposed restraint and imperative, every lifestyle mantra and sacred duty, every nagging gotta, gotta, gotta as mere commodities of belief. Stroll down the supermarket aisles of life and spend your existential capital on whatever you think will deliver the goods, understanding that *you* chose it.

For it is one thing to stave off entropy and fight back the onrushing tide of eternity, cringing by the fire in your cave hoping that bears won't eat you while you sleep, it is another thing entirely to walk into the light and choose life.

MORTAL TERROR THROUGH A RISK / REWARD PRISM

As previously indicated, this book is endeavouring to co-opt the conceptual kitbag of economics to help you develop a different way of thinking about life issues, so rather than continue further along the tunnel of Existentialism and armchair physics let's switch back to our risk/reward mechanism.

Whatever its flaws, economics is a good deal more honest about uncertainty than virtually anything on offer in the various spiritual traditions; especially when we strip out the moral and social ideologies that sometimes warp the narrower schools of economic thought. Indeed, the risk/reward analytical approach, with its emphasis on ascertaining probable outcomes and its inherent admission that every possible win contains a measure of loss, is well suited to a more pragmatic evaluation of our life choices. In other words, it creates a framework whereby we might sift and sort behaviour and choice patterns without necessarily being nailed to a cross of shoulds.

Thus, whilst we can only speculate about ultimate truths and post-death states, as a species we obviously remain certain enough about our mortality to have developed cultures and philosophies rooted in the fear of it. So, given that we pretty well universally accept the fact of death (the end of the current 'I') there are two clear strategies for dealing with it: be afraid or be unafraid.

My bet is that, currently, you are far more likely to belong to the school of the former, if not consciously then almost certainly unconsciously. It is, after all, the evolved norm. So, let's examine some of the costs and benefits of the ubiquitous 'fear of death' position.

Upsides:

- Informs a desire to be fit & healthy – prudent self-care, etc.
- Underpins a potentially motivating sense of urgency – time is running out.
- Occasionally motivates exceptional 'against all odds' perseverance – miracle survival feats.
- Can motivate a desire to leave something of lasting value behind – a glorious legacy – works of art – cures for disease – improved social justice outcomes for others, etc.

Downsides:

- Places fear at or near the very centre of motivation – thereby underpinning 'safety first' and 'me first' positions.
- Underpins a vulnerability to threats – you have something you really are terrified of losing – if you don't, I'll kill you, etc.

- Underpins a vulnerability to painful compromise – kill her, not me – oh well, I had no choice – sell out beliefs and other people, etc.
- Makes you more susceptible to spiritual blackmail – karma and other ethical obedience narratives – eternal damnation.
- Makes you susceptible to medical blackmail – have this expensive and invasive treatment – get addicted to this basket of pharmaceuticals – be a bedwetting, mush-eating prisoner in this nursing home for years on end, etc.
- Makes you more likely to be obedient – the enforcement of rules is, after all, predicated on the believable threat and visible exercise of punishment.
- Makes you more likely to adopt unduly risk-averse positions – fear-based, overly conservative choices – oh, I'd better not, etc.
- Drives absurd vanity projects, monumentalist excess and shallow fame seeking – must get star on pavement – must be the greatest ever – leave big vulgar tomb and/or dynastic legacy, etc.
- Drives a desire to take up gym memberships and kale smoothie consumption – give up fun and undergo all manner of ordeals in an ultimately futile pursuit.

At the end of the day, having a dark seam of overarching dread running through the centre of your life strikes me not only as utterly ineffective (because all the mortal terror in the world won't save you) but likely to render you prone to all manner of externally ordained imperatives and threats of punishment (human or otherwise).

Given that your existential reserve currency (time) is steadily dwindling you have to wonder what the value proposition of the death fear actually is. I mean, what is the pay-off again?

Conversely, a more phlegmatic position seems more likely to serve you better – not in the hereafter perhaps but in this life you're living now. The elimination or drastic reduction of fear allows you the freedom of the 'nothing to lose' position. Making choices that *aren't* underpinned by fear is, I think, plainly a better option.

To state it in stark and extreme terms, it would be much more difficult to put the frighteners on someone who wasn't afraid to die.

In addition, the alleged 'rewards' of the mortal dread strategy are not off limits to those of us with a more casual approach to finality. Just because I'm not afraid to die doesn't mean I won't demonstrate prudent self-care, persevere against the odds or strive to leave something good behind for others to benefit from.

NB:

Indeed, in Chapter 9 – Ethical Investment In A Meaningless Void – I discuss the reasons to be a 'moral actor', even when nothing actually matters.

To be fair though, being cool with ephemerality doesn't preclude vanity, being a sell out or indulging in the conspicuous consumption of this year's must eat superfood. Nor indeed does it prevent enlightenment smugness, callous disregard for one's fellow human beings or any other grave character flaws or modes of idiocy you care to list.

Ultimately, I'm not here to suggest that no longer being scared of dying will make you a 'better' person – just happier, more carefree and at greater liberty to make the choices and follow the paths that *you* select.

Given that the universe is way beyond our total comprehension, and indeed that the observable universe is most likely only a fraction of the actual universe, finding a mechanism that truly increases your likelihood of greater happiness appears to me at least to be eminently sensible. Furthermore, if that mechanism can be employed without cruelty to others or placing undue pressure on yourself, much the better, I say.

So, just as you were not afraid of the void *before* you were born, why be in fear of the one to come after? In fact, the more you genuinely examine the fear of death the more absurd it seems. It's manifestly futile, potentially debilitating, and renders you prone to parental/external blackmail narratives that wedge you into the pursuit of crap that mostly leaves you frustrated, miserable and feeling like a failure.

Sorry to go on about it, but really … isn't it time we all just lived instead?

6.
THE EMANCIPATION EQUATION

or

A bunch of reasons to take the risk and be free

In short, when we drill right down, power and the folk who exercise it are resented, if not demonised; this despite the fact that almost all of us would gladly accept a position of rank, wealth and influence were it offered.

In this chapter I outline the reasons to be free; by which I mean operating in the belief that you are free to self-author more fully and are not compelled, unduly restrained or oppressed by external forces. Furthermore, I examine the link between feeling at liberty and taking responsibility and investigate the cost/benefit of victimhood.

Freedom. It's a fine sounding idea. In the West we cherish it as a foundation stone of our current social contract – the idea that we are all inherently equal and free to live the lives we wish to, providing that our pursuit of life, liberty and happiness doesn't unduly harm others along the way. To what extent this ideal maps out in the real world is debatable. For just as there are conservatives who think that all meaningful social justice battles have been either effectively won or are examples of PC gone mad, there are lefties and conspiracists who claim that we are living in a sinister dystopia where freedom is an illusion built upon the distracting spectacles of consumerism and infotainment.

However, my intention here isn't to dissect either of these ideologies as a socio-political doctrine but to reflect upon the power of these and other beliefs in our personal lives. As indicated in Chapter 4, there are countless should and/or slave narratives out there and all of them offer their believers three key benefits.

- Reduces complexity, ambiguity and uncertainty to generally simple assertions – neatly encapsulates the mess and noise of life and the universe, thus rendering it safer and more readily navigable.
- Externalises responsibility – creating ready-made excuses for poor behaviour and/or passivity – establishes an external authority complex to which to defer – delineates a more easily defined enemy against which to impotently rage.

    +

- Provides a source of external validation – legitimises your choices – underwrites your beliefs.

Freedom, on the other hand, dispenses no such palliatives. Indeed, liberty's sibling is responsibility. The truly free are the ultimately responsible. They do not abdicate accountability to personalised deities, karmic assessment panels or military/industrial complexes. They seek neither the approval of a parental/external authority or the perverse, passive-aggressive emotional drama of the sinner/victim.

To put it less technically – freedom allows you to claim the credit but asks that you be prepared to accept the blame.

This sounds almost ridiculously straightforward. Just an obvious part of being adult. So why do so many of us continue to invest in systems of belief about the world and ourselves that cast us as existential toddlers clinging to the apron strings of a supposedly loving yet always quick to punish external mandation complex?

At least partly, this can be explained by the way in which we first come to know the world and ourselves – or the I and the Not I. As children we learn that our parents (and to a lesser extent other authority figures) not only offer love, nourishment and reward but impose limits using rules we can't quite understand and punishments we soon learn to fear. Later, as parents, we re-administer this medicine, believing all the while that our love is unconditional. Indeed, that may well be our honest intention but to the child the goodies are always purchased with obedience. Only good little girls and boys get treats.

My intention here is not to criminalise the universal routines of parenting; after all, as social animals we are reared in a world that requires prudent curbs on individual action. The entire edifice of morality is structured around this fact. Highly evolved and nuanced ethical behaviour is a brilliant group survival strategy that enables otherwise desirous and self-seeking creatures capable of ingeniously organised cruelty and violence to extract lasting benefits from the synergies of herd cohesion.

However, the notion of conditionality – be good, get rewarded – isn't, in my view, sufficient to explain the plethora of ways in which fully grown adults submit themselves to all manner of shoulds, musts and 'got no choices'. Or indeed, to consciously argue for their own enslavement to patriarchies, central banking cabals and all manner of dominant paradigms.

In Chapter 4 I examined what I call the narrative palliative – that edge-dulling, disambiguating, reductionist morphine of storybook explanation that persists in adult populations everywhere – but here I want to tease apart a couple of the common conceptual habits that bind so many of us in child-like dependency.

In doing so I will clearly be speaking both from (and mostly to) the perspective of the contemporary West; for here in the liberal individual free world slave narratives are everywhere.

THE FALLACY OF SYSTEM

The System. We've all heard of it, spoken of it, felt ripped off, wronged and hemmed in by it. Conversely, most of us have also endeavoured to exploit it in our favour. It is, we tell ourselves, an inevitable part of our lives. Whichever ism we apply, whatever name or frame we use to describe it, and regardless of how we elect to fight against it, we have convinced ourselves, culturally and individually, that it exists.

Yet when we drill into this 'system thing' we discover certain qualities that are common across its numerous incarnations.

- It is essential – as though woven into the background fabric of things – it's been here for ever, or at least for ages – it's unavoidable – the natural order of things, etc.

- It is machine-like – it operates with a grinding, mechanistic inevitability that overrides mere individuals, sometimes even those at the top – it is a rule-based function – cold, ruthless, programmatic, etc.

- It is monolithic – it is the way, the order of things – even apparently divergent 'ways' are really part of its continuing operation – it has a totalitarian and/or omnipresent quality.

- It utilises an invisible hand – it is secretive, covert – a sinister puppet master or a benign but mysterious deity.

- It insists upon your obedience – legality and associated enforcement/punishment mechanisms – inducements in the form of eternal life or Earthly reward in return for compliance – render unto Caesar and, hey presto, bread & circuses, etc.

In addition, many of the most popular system models have an in-built and forever imminent apocalypse. Jesus may be a tad overdue but rest assured He's not far off now. Various days of judgement, atonement and reckoning are already pencilled in. The Caliphate is nigh. The Jewish/Bolshevik international banking conspiracy will soon be revealed. The lizards will be unmasked. Our under siege pineal glands will soon awaken from their fluoridated slumber to herald the dawn of a new golden age. *Viva le revolucion!*

Whether it's the result of destiny, despotism or divine scheming, The System brings overwhelming force to the table; a force that reduces the individual to a cog, a pawn, an actor. At best, a child in God's grade school; the barefoot novice struggling on the rocky lower slopes of a seemingly endless slog up the Everest of nirvana. At worst, little more than a slave.

Therefore, in the shadow of this almighty behemoth it's perfectly acceptable to yield meekly to the way of things, or even to protest loudly whilst nonetheless capitulating – and of course to keep up a grumbling narrative of resentment, complaint and blame.

Hence, my pithy assertion: system blaming is the engine of passivity.

However, in my view, there is something even more remarkable about the so-called system; namely, that it doesn't actually exist.

Okay, so at a 'whole of universe' level I can't be *absolutely 100% sure* that there isn't a divine plan for me, or that some extra-cosmic conscious entity hasn't intelligently designed the exquisitely mathematical jewel that is the cosmos in order to realise some alpha-plan for something that I will never fully comprehend but … a) given the paucity of evidence for such a thing and, b) the high likelihood that such notions are anthropogenic, wishful thinking projections, it seems a better bet for me to believe that the only universal imperatives I am bound to obey are the same ones that govern atoms, gamma rays and the catalysation of proteins. While this is evidence of a highly ordered, gloriously beautiful, supremely elegant system, it has no favourites. It is not moral, nor is it political, even if it *is* as mechanically deterministic as some models suggest. It does not exalt or vilify me because I'm straight, male, Anglo-Saxon and able to ingest gluten at will. I am neither its victim nor its hero – and I am most certainly not 'entitled' by it.

Back down here on the everyday human/social scale though, The System is only 'real' because we make it so. Indeed, system is just another word for custom, for standard practise, for business as usual. The cold, impersonal machinery of government isn't impersonal at all – in fact, it's made entirely *of* people (computerisation and algorithms notwithstanding). Every rule bound, process driven decision is made by an individual or groups of individuals in consultation; and even if precedent, prejudice, penny pinching and 'computer says no' *do* play their part, and grossly unfair outcomes result from this, it is still the upshot of *human* action.

Quite simply, government, economy, the law, science, academia and religion are all human institutions. Our habit of externalising and dehumanising these activities, reducing them to monolithic system narratives, lets both perpetrator and victim off the hook of accountability. All the while we humans regard system as the other we will continue in a slave relationship with it.

Yet, when we prise apart the structure of the various system models what we discover are simply patterns of repeated behaviour. We can call them received wisdoms or isms if we wish but the description doesn't alter the basic underlying fact. System is habit.

In saying this I am in no way seeking to minimise or deny the existence of cruelty, injustice, oppression, exploitation, entrenched privilege or the essentialisation of out groups. These are sadly frequent human traits. The list of our nasty, stupid and destructive customs is long – and all of them are enshrined and enacted through the agency of individual and group choice. Each act of violence is just that, an *act*. It's *people* who are responsible for this shit – not systems. Not the machines we've invented or the Gods we made up. It's us. Folks remarkably like you, dear reader.

You may, at this point, once again be saying 'yeah, so what, that's obvious' and my response would similarly be 'yeah, I know, but …' And the 'but' in this case would be that, despite this indisputable fact, many of us continue to relate to The System not as something that humans *choose* but as though it were a kind of immutable law. We have successfully separated The System from ourselves, casting it as an externality, a nigh abstract and essential function. As for the people who work for (or in) The System we have delineated them as an out group. Politicians, merchant bankers, media magnates, members of the Rothschild and Windsor families and even faceless bureaucrats are routinely considered nefarious, stupid or corrupt. Indeed, even those who are employed by governments, banks and television stations are wont to rail against the heartless, moronic, pocket lining 'higher ups' who make their lives a misery. As a consequence, the notion of system allows us to dehumanise one another along inside/outside lines.

In short, when we drill right down, power and the folk who exercise it are resented, if not demonised; this despite the fact that almost all of us would gladly accept a position of rank, wealth and influence were it offered, and may actually be working assiduously towards such a goal even as I type. Indeed, many of us probably believe we would make excellent world rulers or CEOs. No wonder so much that commonly passes for dissent is little more than envy rebadged or infantile 'it's not fair' dummy spitting. Observe the endless slurry of simplistic populist outcry that parades as common sense solution or people power on talkback radio, Facebook feeds or in the pages of Murdoch-owned tabloids. (The irony of all these whinge-friendly platforms being operated by mega-corporations and funded by evil banking cartels is clearly lost on the so-called 99%.)

Whilst it's entirely understandable that we don't enjoy feeling powerless or relish the fact that decisions we have little or no say in may adversely affect us, our belief in so-called systems dulls the pain of this by allowing us to convince ourselves that our helplessness is an inevitable corollary of history, destiny or fiendishly hatched conspiracy. This then leaves us free to blame The System for the fact that we find ourselves living lives that don't bring us joy and pursuing objectives that we don't really believe in. After all, it is easier to be a whinging infant bemoaning the unfair restrictions of the parental/external than it is to accept full adult responsibility. Simpler to be an almost blameless slave than free to own up.

Of course, in saying this I do wish to distinguish between those living with genuine poverty and oppression, or in war zones, and those currently residing in the beige comfort of middle class suburbia. The seventeen-year-old girl being married off to the dirty old fucker who raped her or the slumdog kids eking out a grubby subsistence from other people's rubbish have a damn sight less wriggle room than the Audi driving, iThing wielding, Netflix subscriber who rails against glass ceilings, political correctness or working too hard.

In the West, where levels of physical wellbeing and security are historically high and where the erosion of once rigid customs has allowed for a far greater social and economic mobility than exists in more traditionally rule bound societies, there is a palpable sense of discontent. The widespread idea that things are fundamentally fucked and that we're all going to hell in a handbasket is evident in phenomena as diverse as the retreat into mawkish, generational nostalgia and expressions of full blown ideological rage against the machine. Whether we're bemoaning the fact that it's no longer acceptable to thrash the children or that modern democracy has devolved into a relentlessly idiotic adversarial spectacle, we have developed countless 'world gone mad' scenarios to imprison ourselves in a slave/master relationship with The System.

Identity politics as a system blaming slave narrative

At the time of writing – circa 2019 – we in the West are enduring the fist-shaking spectacle of so-called identity politics. In this mode of polemic paranoia, the believer typically casts themselves as being specifically and deliberately victimised because of their nominated identity (woman/man, white/black, gay/straight, etc). This victimisation is routinely regarded as systemic and in its theoretical construction it involves simplistic us/them, good/bad dichotomies which dehumanise the 'other' and infer upon the in group an almost naturally occurring moral, biological and/or cultural superiority. In addition, the identity mantra is often rooted in entitlement and, of course, in 'poor me' thinking. As with conspiracy, identity politics invokes both the poison world view and a self-attributed victim status to give it emotional urgency, missionary zeal and the satisfying fizz of righteous rage. The best we can say about Western identity politics in the Trump Era is that it's undergraduate; although I regard it as closer to infantile. That our polity and cultural discourse has devolved into a junior school shout-off, with the various sides yelling dumb slogans at one another over the airwaves, underscores this retraction into the easy comforts of childish certitude and illustrates just how pervasive system blaming slave-think is.

All the while we cling onto beliefs that tell us that we *have* to get a steady job, upgrade the phone or wax our genitals to a pre-pubescent shine, we are effectively talking ourselves into a state of helplessness. The System doesn't so much force us to obey, as we prop up The System with our continued obedience.

In short – and perhaps somewhat brutally – what I'm suggesting here is that blaming the so-called system for your unhappiness, resentment and sense of incarceration is disingenuous at best. You are not, in fact, a slave – you're just addicted to the idea that you are and, if you're honest, you get a perverse kick from the righteous thrill it gives you. Poor, noble me battling quixotically against the numerous evils of the poison world. And look, here my chains, here my badges of honour. (Here my cast iron excuses.)

Thus, in order to dilute that beloved victim narrative, we need to wean ourselves from the breast milk of systems – from the apparent inevitabilities of the parental/external – and to view the social world (culture, politics, economy, etc) as human and not as some kind of abstract mechanism. Our societies are behavioural, and it is with our personal contributions that we either bolster the status quo or offer up alternatives.

Once we come to think of cold dystopian machinery as simply the result of human choices – behaviour – the overwhelming nature of system power dissolves. In this light it becomes clear that we can no longer continue in system blame, or indeed to recognise The System as something that exists outside of us. Indeed, when we disavow ourselves of the multitude of externalised power complexes and the Essentialist imperatives they uphold we can begin to regard ourselves as the true source of power in our lives. For better or worse. Now we are finally ready to be free.

THE WANT / NEED PROBLEM

If system narratives are all about establishing an abstract edifice of external validation and compulsion, the want/need problem is avowedly personal. It is also virtually universal. Along with pretty well everyone I have ever met, I too have fallen into the trap of confusing want with need.

However, it is also one of the easiest shackles to unlock; not least because, intellectually, it's a no brainer. Quite clearly,

---

The waning of want

From personal experience, what I have noticed with want (desire) is that in most cases it is temporary. It passes. Generally, it is stimulated in proximity to its object – i.e. I feel like chocolate when I'm looking at it in the shop. However, I have observed that desire mostly evaporates shortly thereafter. (Often, even if I carry the chocolate in the basket, my desire for it wanes before I get to the checkout and now, most of the time, I end up putting it back on the shelf – not because I'm a good boy or nobly denying myself pleasure but because I've realised that I don't *really* want it.) The pay-off here is the everyday, lived experience of *not* being a slave to my desires and, what's more, that the physical and emotional urgencies of wanting will wane over time (minutes usually) and create the opportunity for more considered choices. I will admit to finding this an empowering phenomenon, one that has fed into a greater sense of self-trust and esteem; and all without dogmatically pathologising my desires and/or lapsing into self-punishment.

NB: I elaborate on similar themes in Chapter 10 – especially in the '15 things' section.

as sentient and gendered social mammals, we do indeed have hardwired physical needs – food, water, shelter, etc – and fundamental psychological needs – loving parent(s), a level of herd acceptance, touch, etc. In addition, the mechanism of sexual reproduction drives a need for pair-bonding intimacy.

Furthermore, within the context of a large super-tribal society (city, province, nation) the goal of meeting these needs and balancing out the competing claims of individuals underwrites the most basic tenets of the social contract and, from there, the broad brushstrokes of our political and economic behaviour and the core values at work in the law.

Yet, once the human animal transitioned from concrete clan-based, co-operative organisation to larger, abstracted societies with greater division and specialisation of labour, we began to create large staple food surpluses and a far greater range of tools, textiles and trinkets. For the first time in our history we had reasonably reliable access to more. Much more. On the back of this, some groups in society began to enjoy extended free time and, along with higher learning and new technologies, they developed a taste for non-essential items like jewellery, status and delicacies.

As agricultural surpluses fed the growth of city states and their empires they also spurred on a huge flowering of trade. Before too long there were luxury items for sale (spices, silks, slaves and so on) and various forms of money with which to buy them.

Alongside this increasing complexity, the further solidification of class stratas and the refinement of skill sets into recognisable 'trades' led to the creation of a dynamic, diversified and dangerous social ecosphere that mimicked our evolved relationship of dependence and struggle with the natural environment. (The urban jungle, no less.)

Thus, as the distance between nature and the world we were busy making for ourselves grew, so too there was a kind of 'socialisation of necessity'. As more and more of us became increasingly blind to the raw physical facts of food provision, and of protecting ourselves from nocturnal carnivores, the focus of our need also shifted from immediate physiological imperative to economic survival; and in turn, the gathering of socially visible trophies of status and the satisfaction of longer term objectives. Indeed, somewhere along the line, pleasures became necessities and luxuries a baseline minimum. Today, we believe we must be experience collectors, or indeed be sexily self-improved. We must *all* be great. We absolutely *have* to kit ourselves out in the latest fashion slacks or be observed to extol the delicious benefits of this season's groovily over-priced and supposedly miraculous ancient grain.

Of course this is ridiculous, a mere capitulation to peer pressure and the marketing mavens who exploit it. You know it as well as I do. I only *want* to be rich, cool and fuckable. Sure, I'd *like* to take a leisurely river cruise past a bunch of French castles or get someone to fund my outrageously indulgent feature film project. Shucks, it would even be sweet if someone published this book for you to buy and read. But *need?* Nope.

Yet for all that, want is mistaken for need in virtually every loungeroom, boardroom and changing room of every human culture. Here in the West we have become culturally convinced that genuine need includes things like smartphone apps, gym memberships and LinkedIn profiles. All around the world, people tell themselves they *need* to cultivate and maintain certain relationships – and so they frequently resort to deference, flattery and tight-lipped obedience and, along the way, effectively tolerate and condone behaviours that are harmful to themselves and others and which, in fact, may even be abusive and predatory.

Maybe it's not too great a stretch to suggest that 'I need to' in these contexts really means something like, 'I don't want to but I believe I have to.' Here again we hear the voice of the slave. The language of abdicated responsibility. Once more the locus of power is externalised and the inculcated narratives of the parental/external are dominant. Even if we submit begrudgingly, it's still submission.

Indeed, I would wager that if you were to run a scan of your apparent needs you would discover that the percentage of *actual* needs amongst them would be quite low. You may also notice that a great number of them are associated with desires and imperatives around status, vanity and entertainment. Things like keeping up appearances, competing with perceived rivals and the fear of missing out on the awesome fun everyone else on Facebook is apparently having. Then, digging deeper still, you may even discover that most of those pesky internal voices telling you that you must do this or ought to be more like that sound strangely like those of parent and authority figures, like partners and family members; and, worryingly, like the more, more, more mantras of advertising or the ideological pestering of those who want you to conform to their particular practise. In other words, voices of external judgement and control.

Recognising the need/want confusion and identifying the externally mandated narratives you've bought into is the first step in effectively disarming their power and taking full responsibility for your choices. For when we learn the trick of sifting out external imperatives from genuinely personal goals we gain the clarity to make honest, informed choices. We are able to take more control because we have jettisoned the 'have to' rationale.

NB:

For more on this, check out Chapter 10, The Authenticity Channel.

Remember, unless someone is actually holding a gun to your head or issuing other believable violent and coercive threats, you never really *have* to. Even then you could just shrug and say, 'go on then, kill me.' Point is: ought and should are almost always excuses. Forms of abdication.

Personally, once I disentangled want from need, I uncovered the power of genuine choice. I still make bad ones but of one thing I am clear: they are mine. Whilst external sources continue to *inform* my choices and I do still accord with a raft of social norms, I do so understanding the risk/reward equation of both concurrence and divergence. Within the context of the contemporary human social world in which I move (and within the confines of biology and physics) I now exercise that thing called freedom. And I love it.

THE TRUE VALUE OF VICTIMHOOD

Of course, you are entirely free to choose slavery. If believing that you're being shat upon by the Bilderberg Group, hoodwinked by the Illuminati or ripped off by either the feminazis or the patriarchy *really* makes you happy, please, polish your chains. Wear them as bling if you wish.

You may well say 'but these things are real' and I would concur that injustice, unfairness and bigotry do indeed exist. Yes, there are zealots in both conservative and progressive camps who take things too far. True, class and caste structures do continue to prop up a largely hereditary few at the expense of the many, and the neo-liberal free market agenda that has predominated since the 1980s has indeed underscored a massive uptick in income disparity and unsustainable resource use. And sure, it is reasonable to hold these things up to scrutiny, if not outright condemnation.

However, there is a big difference between well-reasoned criticism (and the active advocacy and/or protest action it can inspire) and mere passive whingeing – and, to be fair, it is the latter that I observe far more of.

I do not believe it unfairly harsh to suggest that the ratio of complaint to action most likely hovers somewhere in the million to one region. Here in the digitally connected West the vast majority of us don't even bother to spend the two minutes it takes to sign online petitions. Indeed, the most active most of us get is to hit Like or Share on Facebook. Very few of us march in the streets or write to MPs, let alone take the time to sift out the facts from the rhetoric or, heaven forfend, contemplate the potential validity of an opposing viewpoint.

Aside from accusing virtually everyone of monumental laziness, there are several commonly advanced reasons (or excuses) for the disconnect between discontent and doing anything about it.

- I'm too busy.
- It won't make any difference, so why bother?
- I'm not into politics.
- Those hairy armpit, femo types are far too puritanical – no bloody fun.
- There's just so much conflicting information out there – who to believe?

Whatever your particular reason is, the point I'm driving at here isn't so much political as personal and psychological. If we break down the above what we arrive at is a sense of helplessness and/or ineffectiveness. It's a form of defeatism. A kind of victim impact statement. *I'm just a poor boy, blah, blah, blah.*

Whereas it is often prudent to admit defeat with equanimity and say 'oh, well, never mind, better luck next time,' it is another to remain in a loop of futility, complaint and conspiracist paranoia. Likewise, whilst it's perfectly fine *not* to take an interest in politics or social justice – or indeed to understand how the economy functions, move to a higher vibration or say no to drugs – it's another to feel victimised by The System, or like a hapless fool who's just not good enough.

Or, to put it another way – on one hand there is calm and considered disengagement and acceptance, on the other there's simmering, impotent discontent, frustration and a crushing, cancerous sense of failure.

You know better than I which of those best describes your current situation.

That said, in my experience, the latter is more common. Even in the well-off, inner city postcode where I live I encounter much more slave-think than free-think. My neighbours may dress fashionably, earn good money and otherwise adopt the look and feel of liberal-progressive sophisticates but still I hear them declaring themselves the poor little victims of everything from white male corporate oppression to the creeping scourge of Shari'a Law. And then there are those who are the mere vessels of destiny – the 'meant to be' drones desperately trying to decipher the universe's arcane plan for them.

The commonality? They are all being done to, as opposed to doing, and if they're not feeling unjustly squeezed by The System they're striving madly to cram for their cosmic/karmic examination by doing what they supposedly 'came here' for.

This would all be fine if they were happy about it – if they weren't straining at their chains. Or indeed if they were content to confess to the cop out. Even *ah well, fuck it, whatever* would be a better option in my view. So, here's where we turn again to our risk/reward prism and ask …

- Does being a victim really pay off for you?
- Is the blame shifting mentality of the slave a better deal than the responsibility of freedom?

Remember, it's okay if you prefer the slave role if it genuinely delivers the goods. It is, as I have said previously, your life to lead.

However, if, as I suspect, that sense of frustration and unfairness, of looming catastrophe, of battling against insurmountable odds, of never quite being up to scratch, of always needing to prove yourself, of never having enough, of feeling that no matter what you do nothing will change for the better … well, you know what I'm gonna say.

Time to consider a different existential investment strategy. Time to take the plunge on freedom. Accept the blame, own the fuck-ups, author the meaning, write the rules, break them at will, and *do whatever you want*.

After all, your life's reserve currency (time) is running out and all the while you are spending this non-recoupable asset on shit you'd rather not be doing with arseholes you can't stand for ends that don't make you happy or inspire you – or you feel like a defenceless cog in a relentless conveyer belt of systematic oppression or an unworthy piece of shit on the sole of God's runners – you are swindling yourself rotten. You may as well go shopping, buy a load of crap you don't like, will never eat or wear outdoors and, to rub a little salt in, pay with it from an expense account that will never be topped up. Then, when you get back home with your trolley load of worthless garbage, berate yourself for being such a tool and wish the fuck you'd bought something else.

Okay, so I've painted the scene somewhat colourfully but I suspect that most of you know what I'm driving at and, if you're honest, will recognise such behaviours in yourself. I have most definitely been guilty of such thinking and, most likely, will relapse into old habits in future times of particular stress and misfortune. It is, after all, only human to feel helpless and/or worthless on occasion – and indeed there *are* external circumstances that we do not control.

However, I have learned the simple but profoundly powerful trick of regarding these travails as episodes rather than as examples of brutalising, paradigmatic inevitability somehow specifically designed to crush me or remind me what a piece of shit I am.

Thus, when I find myself thinking there's a big pattern at work I begin by trying to identify whether the pattern is truly mine (habituated behaviours, familiar self-talk, etc) or indeed stems from the external. Most subsequently turn out to be mine; but even when I *do* conclude that the pattern is external – and maybe even cruel or unjust – I resist the temptation to morph this realisation into an overarching world view that paints me as a powerless speck in a pre-determined, oligarchic mechanism impelling me with uncaring hands towards the clifftop of apocalypse.

Your local cut/copy conspiracist will doubtless suggest that I'm kidding myself, that I'm just another one of the shopping mall sheeple being herded by the puppeteers of the New World Order. Here again, rather than simply asserting that they're wrong, let's borrow from the economist's conceptual toolkit, remind ourselves of a few key points, turn our focus to matters of utility and uncertainty, and run the risk metrics in order to ascertain the true existential value of victimhood.

- Given that I know with absolute certainty that I'm going to die at some unknown point in the future, I therefore place great value on my steadily decreasing stockpile of days and nights and thus on my potential to extract the maximum amount of beauty, meaning, etc, from this remaining time.

- I also know that regardless of how clever, moral, right/wrong or otherwise I think I am, and no matter what marvellous achievements or howling failures I rack up, I will be just as dead as everyone else – saint, sinner, superstar, et al. Any accumulated status, apparent wisdom or tally of so-called musts I've ticked off the list will count for nothing in the final hour.

- Unless the NSA, the Wahhabists or some angry deity determine that I really must be killed right now, the opinions and objectives of others or the whims of gods will almost certainly *not* affect the timing or manner of my demise – meaning that the power of external, socially imposed narratives and judgements about how I should live have very little *actual* clout. In fact, aside from matters of law and a few truly exceptional circumstances (like being raped or tortured), the only power they have over me is the power I invest in them.

- Therefore, even if I am being manipulated by the 1% or railroaded by destiny – and indeed free will itself is a delusion – I am still left with an amount of time to fill and with the power to maintain, alter or abandon my beliefs about both myself and the wider world. Delusional or not, I remain at liberty to select my beliefs (narratives, worldviews, tropes, etc) from a spectrum that runs from the pleasant and empowering 'fantasy' of freedom and genuine authorship to the doomful, rat-in-a-box, 'only doin' it cos I have to' disposition of the self-shackling slave.

- Meanwhile, at the metaphysical or spiritual level, it seems only fair that I admit a modicum of uncertainty around the existence or otherwise of gods, Essentialist meanings and their associated imperatives. After all, given my clearly limited perspective and capacity, to declare *absolute* certainty here would border on fundamentalist arrogance and I therefore accept that what remains is belief. (Or faith if you prefer.) And so, down here at the level of the quantised self I am still, as I said above, left to orient myself through a world for an ever-shortening amount of time and thus, to find the most conducive and rewarding method of travel. In this regard, as a mortal primate, notions of ultimate truth border on practical irrelevance – even if they do make for excellent red wine conversation and find their way into books like this. In conclusion, the ongoing function of any beliefs I may hold in this area will map out in my daily living as either adding to and enriching my experience, or not. Why then, would I choose to think of myself as an unworthy acolyte, repetitively failing nirvana candidate or bit part player in some pre-planned drama about whatever the fuck?

- In the end the experience of being *me* (of the current and particular self-conscious identity event I recognise as my life here on Earth) will stop, and any fussing I may do about being cool, rich, successful or part of an enlightened elite will have amounted, in the final analysis, to zero. Any observance of customs, tolerating of fuckwits and tyrants, or sense of being oppressed by whichever nasty cohort I care to identify will have got me precisely nowhere.

- Indeed, in strict existential utility terms, even being right or wrong is a less significant distinction than the choice between having a sense of agency and control or believing that I'm a hard done by victim who just isn't good enough.

As I am wont to bore my friends by saying, I would much rather be a screaming failure at what I love than a success at what I hate. Along with a reduction in the desire for peer approval or socially visible status, and a parallel de-coupling from the striving mantra so ingrained in our culture, this mindset has effectively handed me the prison keys. I can come and go as I please now.

The pay-offs of the slave mentality just do not compare.

STATUS OBJECTS & SILVER BULLETS

Like me, you have probably met the alt-poser; that person at the party who wears the badge that says 'awakened'. This person exalts and professes their own rebellious superiority and seems to be very keen for you to understand that patriarchal, Judeo-Christian norms just don't apply in their case.

Of course, we both know that this is the likeness of freedom as a status seeking spectacle. *Allow me to place my enlightened penis inside you. Please deposit fifteen hundred dollars into my highly vibrating bank account. Crawl to the altar of my non-sexist, macrobiotic, ethically sourced, dairy free, shamanically revealed higher purpose.*

My point here is not to mock the idea of fair trade or to denigrate the shamanic tradition, or even to suggest that charging for counselling or healing is inherently wrong, but to draw an important distinction. Because when freedom is a boast it's not really freedom. It's really still centred on drawing favourable attention to yourself and/or delineating oneself from 'the masses' in order to feel somehow special or anointed.

You may well accuse me of doing this now – and indeed I confess to being at least partly conflicted by the action of writing this book. I mean, why do I care if you understand my point of view or are convinced by my arguments? Couldn't I just quietly bumble along in my own minimalist, Existentialist, ecstatically nihilistic way without resorting to the pomposity of philosophy? And the answer is yes. Of course I could.

The other thing I could do at this point is to indulge in a bout of white, middle class guilt. You know the kind of thing: shame on me for drawing attention to myself, for having the arrogance to think that my ideas and experiences might be in any way interesting to others. However, this would simply be punitive, self-lacerating judgement based on a moral narrative that I am not genuinely convinced by. It would also be a pose, if not for others then for myself.

In the end it turns out that lasting, enjoyable, practical freedom pivots not only upon our attitude towards the external but in making a kind of peace with the internal. For what is the use of liberty if it doesn't help you to live a more enriched and rewarding life? If being free becomes just another must on a bucket list of compulsory attainment its pursuit will soon morph into either a rod of punishment – *oh no, I'm not free enough* – or an approval seeking bauble of fashionable enlightenment.

Freedom doesn't mean you're superior or wise. It does not offer to extend your life or get you laid, neither will it necessarily fatten your finances, get your book published or render all your actions pure. Furthermore, it gives you no guarantee that suicide bombers, traffic accidents or seismic activity won't wipe you out. Indeed, it won't even stop you being unhappy.

Rather, freedom simply puts an existential proposition on the table. Its risk/reward calculus goes something like this:

- If you can let go of stuff like the 'have to' excuse and the must list, outgrow the baby food mush of easy answers and accept with equanimity the relative insignificance of your own existence and the equalising and extinguishing fact of your death, then you will be free to live. Truly live – as you genuinely choose. For the sheer beauty of it.

And who knows, you might even choose to write a book about it. Not because you think it will get hot bodies beating down your bedroom door or win you brownie points with Krishna but just because you enjoy it. Because getting to the end of this chapter will feel really good; and the coffee you will make yourself right after the final full stop will taste bloody wonderful.

7.
THE BELIEF BRIEF

or

The power of not really believing too much of anything

Once we can surrender the idea that we have to
work everything out, that the right belief
will lead us to some kind of jackpot, we realise
that to a large extent it simply doesn't matter
what we believe.

In this chapter I pose questions like: do your beliefs serve you or do you serve them? In addition, I argue that not having too many beliefs and not believing stuff too strongly (dogmatically) will make for a much less stressful, far more flexible and noticeably 'lighter' life. After all, surely our beliefs should contribute to our wellbeing, as opposed to enslaving us.

Before we go any further, let's remind ourselves why we're here. (Why I'm indoors writing on a pleasantly warm spring afternoon and you're still reading.) It's called happiness. Or, if you'd rather:

- Joy
- Contentment
- Fulfilment
- Wellbeing

Or even:

- A deeper sense of meaning

As previously suggested, what I mean by happiness is not mere fun or wild, adrenalised excitement. Nor do I mean enlightenment, purity or perfection. What I'm pointing at is something deep, broadly based and ongoing. This condition doesn't exclude episodes of melancholy or disappointment, nor even of anger, failure and poor decision making. This happiness is not a utopia but a space where you can act with a sense of genuine liberty, empowered to direct your own life for reasons and purposes that *you* have authentically chosen. In other words, where the life you are leading right now more closely resembles the one you hoped for than the one you feel you have to. Perhaps not perfect but certainly getting there.

Indeed, the very reason I am choosing to write this book is because I have come upon this place and I now know how good it is. I also know that I didn't get here because I won a lottery, downloaded a divine secret or ticked fifty seven things off a bucket list. My journey to this point was riddled with wrong turns, false starts, poor choices and no small measure of despair, self-destructive patterns and flat out laziness. I can also confess to ignorance, conceit, complacency and wanton disregard. Yet, flawed as I am, I got here.

So, without lionising myself or extolling my intelligence, strength of character or superior value set, I arrived in this moment of happiness thanks to an often serendipitous journey of trial and error – via an accumulative process of sifting and sorting. I mention this because it underlines the fact that creating the life you want – that doing what you want with your remaining time – does not involve miraculous transformative revelation or heroic visionary capacity. Neither does it require hair shirt abstinence, rigorous spiritual practise or having shedloads of cash. Or, for that matter, reading this book.

What it *does* require is a conscious determination to take honest responsibility and the awareness and discipline to practise putting that decision into action. This involves recognising where your power lies and what things you *can* change and, conversely, acknowledging what you can't affect and will most likely never ever know. In other words, a psycho-emotional and intellectual balancing act – fighting some battles whilst walking away from others. Learning to execute this without punitive self-judgement and attainment mania, and without seeking the dubious status trophies of so-called wisdom, is crucial not only to sustaining the effort and focus needed to keep going but in recognising and disentangling yourself from old personal patterns and external validation cravings.

In saying this though, I also think it's fair to acknowledge 'circumstance'. The arrogant, solipsistic New Age manifestation mantra (the whole universe is a reflection of me and is somehow there to grant my wishes, if only I ask it nicely) is, in my opinion, little more than pseudo-spiritual narcissism, and a grandiose self-centrism that borders on hubris. A kind of neo-liberalism for the greedy soul that reduces the cosmos to a shopping mall.

Hating the West

Nowadays – at least in my circles of association – it is almost *de rigeur* to be hyper-critical of the West. You know the drum – horrible Anglo-Europeans (men mostly) are responsible for all the bad stuff and, remarkably, everything Asian, African, tribal and ancient is automatically wiser, healthier and cooler. In my view, this is a narrative of guilt and self-loathing and is, mostly, a diaphanously righteous pose. Whilst it is reasonable to argue that Western military, economic and cultural imperialism has devastated and distorted the lives and livelihoods of hundreds of millions across the centuries (and often in a repugnantly racist and rapacious fashion), it is surely a misnomer to gloss over the multiple cruelties and prejudices of other civilisations. Our whole *species* is hierarchic, violent and acquisitive, and the very form of what we call 'civilisation' has been inherently unequal since we first began to acquire specialised skills in the aftermath of agriculture and fixed settlement. What's more, we are *all* prone to chauvinism against nominated out groups. Thus, for historically wealthy, healthy and leisured Westerners like myself to maintain a fashionable veneer of auto-disgust, whilst simultaneously enjoying the largesse of welfare states, hot showers and the internet, is disingenuous at best – flat out hypocritical and indulgent at worst. It not only represents a serious loss of perspective but smacks of exactly the kind of self-absorbed laziness and arrogance that anti-Western zealots use as justification for their sometimes murderous activities. In this time in the West we are indeed, as my dad likes to say, the winners of history – and whilst we are right to call out injustice, I think it also behoves us to acknowledge the extreme good fortune of our current socio-economic and cultural environment.

Therefore, to use my own example, it's prudent (even respectful) to acknowledge that a key contributor to my currently happy condition is the fact that I had the luck to be born at a time and into a socio-economic environment that has allowed me the scope for the aforementioned hithering and thithering. I have not been bombed out of house and home, subjected to famine or dragged off to a gulag for publically espousing anti-establishment opinions. Furthermore, I have benefitted from prevailing conditions which have made it possible for a legally blind* man from a working class migrant background to get a tertiary education and live in reasonable physical comfort despite his bohemian proclivities and stop/start career.

(* I was only recently diagnosed as legally blind – in August 2017, not long before I began drafting this chapter.)

Here again, this is to emphasise that my happiness is not the result of some particular and exceptional genius, and also to suggest that the sense of discontent and slave-thinking so common in the contemporary West is at least partly rooted in a staggering loss of perspective and, dare I say, a serious lack of gratitude.

Putting aside the obviously positive effects of gratitude for a moment, a 'sense of perspective' is, I believe, a critical underpinning factor in releasing ourselves from the stranglehold of externally ordained imperatives.

Why do I say this? Well, apart from allowing you a sense of distance from things (from the drama, from the clutter of details) it can also melt down notions of self-importance and soften the edge of so-called certainties; and since so many socially and ideologically mandated assertions are couched in absolutist and/or Essentialist terms, doubt and humility effectively erode the foundations of *you should*, *I must* and *we have no choice*. All of those apparently game critical imperatives and/or abdications to a higher power are really just the reinforcement of common practise – the 'say so' of others on repeat – and though they may at times have genuine merit and serve a good practical purpose they are, after all, just *beliefs*. They may seem important, crucial even, in the hurly burly of our struggle for wealth, status and sexual approval, but viewed from a certain distance they soon recede into relative trivia, becoming mere habits. The mirror-loop of conformity. The symphony of our sweetly clanking chains. The baubles of our vanity.

Yet for all that, I would wager that most of you have already experienced the so-called 'wider perspective' on a number of occasions; so once again, no need for expensive gurus or Himalayan mountaintop retreats. Indeed, it would seem that the real trick is to keep this higher perspective somewhere near the 'front of mind'. Trite as it sounds to say things like *this too shall pass* and *don't take yourself too seriously*, these easily disposable clichés can help to sharpen your focus on the edifice of your beliefs; and get you asking questions like:

- Why do I believe this stuff?
- Is this drama/reason/habit/assertion *really* important?
- Are these truly *my* beliefs or have I simply accepted them as read?
- Do these beliefs serve me … or do I serve them?

For instance, whenever I find myself mired in the 'dailies', bogged down in the details, all my beliefs seem truer and my objectives appear to be genuinely important. *Stuff matters*. In this space I am far more likely to act out of habit, repeat well-worn narratives to myself and accept the presence and ill-treatment of tyrants and other abusers. (Not to mention being a snarky, elitist prick.)

And then I remember to step back and … bam! My beliefs, and the patterned responses they drive, are once more held up to the light. Apparent certainties are revealed again to be oft-recited stories. Obligations become genuine choices. The stubbornness or aggrandisement of my ego dissolves into a sense of relaxed equanimity. Must haves get easily left behind.

For example, I understand clearly that I could stop writing this book at any moment and it wouldn't really matter a jot; for although I like the idea of being the kind of person who has the discipline and focus to see complex projects through to a satisfying conclusion, I only cling to that belief and invest my existential capital in it because it delivers the goods in terms of happiness. (A present and palpable feeling state.) In the end, if it ever becomes apparent that a happier strategy would be to consign the files to the recycle bin, then I will be free to do so without the flagellating spectacle of work ethic narratives or any of those droning, internalised, moralising monologues about perseverance and *having* to.

From where I sit – i.e. the happiest I've ever been – this strikes me as a very profitable bargain with belief. On the whole it now seems that the fewer things I believe and the less strongly I hold onto the beliefs that *do* remain, the happier, calmer, more balanced and less prone to external shocks and social pressure I am.

All of which prompts me to ask: *what are beliefs for?*

Sure, a bunch of them are rooted in basic survival – physical, emotional, social, etc – but that's not what I'm seeking to address here. I'm not questioning the fact that hurling yourself off a seventy-two storey building will result in your grisly and immediate death, nor indeed am I suggesting that you try to exempt yourself from the laws of physics by plastering affirmations to that effect on the back of your bedroom door. What I *am* suggesting is that you ask yourself the aforementioned question with regards to the plethora of socially received, morally loaded, marketing driven, ideologically approved, complacently unexamined, culturally biased, celebrity anointed, swami sanctioned, internet rumoured, media mandated beliefs that all of us are prey to. Things like:

- How to live the bestest, coolest, sexiest, wealthiest, spiritually superior life.*
- How to be a better person – more this, less that, etc.
- I am the way I am because … and so therefore – my right – my punishment – my excuse, etc.
- This is my lot in life, my destiny, my proper function, etc.
- This is what I'm entitled to and you better not try take it from me – fortress mentality.
- I'm being oppressed because I'm …
- These people are role models … but them folks is horrible, thieving motherfuckers.
- Everything's going to shit – doom, gloom, decadence and decay.
- The Muslim, Asian, central banking robot queers are taking over – dystopian future.
- It's the Australian/Ukrainian/Azerbaijani way – nationalist, ethnic and sectarian tropes.

- They don't write songs like that anymore – generational clichés and legislated nostalgia.

(***** Yes, I am aware of the inherent self-contradiction in this; so let's just add blatant hypocrisy to that list of grievous character flaws I mentioned earlier.)

If you are walking around with a bunch of these beliefs, how do they make you feel about yourself, your life and the world? Where on the spectrum do you sit with regards to feeling autonomous or feeling impelled and constrained? Are you stocking up the bunker to ride out the apocalypse? Ring fencing your castle to stop social justice warriors confiscating your *Barely Legal* videos? Going on yet another diet? Social media feeds giving you a bad case of 'fomo'? Still not suitably enlightened? (Oh dear.)

All levity and colourful language aside, ask yourself what on Earth is the point of a belief system and associated mindset that leaves you feeling powerless, envious and unworthy; or like your best days are in the past? On the flipside, are your beliefs about being a worthy winner or a member of some exceptional and specially endowed clique, class or culture also fuelling a hyper-vigilant dread of losing your entitlements to either the mob or to your covetous, conniving cohorts?

In other words, do beliefs of this nature contribute to or detract from your potential happiness?

MAKING THE PORTFOLIO PAY

Returning to our book's subtitle – *The Economics Of Doing Whatever You Want* – we can now adopt a way of examining the existential value of our beliefs without the caveats of external mandation and Essentialist dogma. As per previous chapters, the prism here is based on risk/reward, with outcomes measured in greater or lesser utility and underwritten by the idea that time is the ultimate unit of account.

Again, while it is prudent to acknowledge that some beliefs are physically, emotionally and socially efficacious and, furthermore, that consistent conceptual frameworks can indeed help us to navigate the world and deal with unforeseens, much of what most of us believe and act upon (and internalise and tell ourselves and others) springs from habit, hearsay, vanity, fear, wishful thinking, nostalgia, anthropomorphisation, the muddling of cause and correlation and the desire for neat either/or encapsulations that bolster our entrenched worldviews.

It is, I think, safe to say that much, if not most, of what we commonly believe is *not* solely based in hard objective truth. However, rather than insist upon a rigid 'all beliefs must be 100% factual' doctrine, what I'm suggesting is that the very *act* of believing – our tendency to overlay the numerous uncertainties with disambiguating leaps of faith and personal preference – means that we *already have* the power and the scope to re-examine whether or not our 'belief portfolio' works for us at a lived experience level, hardcore physical/biological truths notwithstanding.

So, whilst purists and ideologues will bang on about truth, morality or divine higher purpose as the motivation for adopting and sticking to a bunch of beliefs, what I'd like to suggest is that happiness is a perfectly adequate reason for investing in a suite of beliefs.

Of course, religious/spiritual types and moral conservatives will scoff, dismissing happiness as trivial in the face of cosmic evolutionary imperatives or God's undergraduate programme for inveterate sinners. At this juncture, it's appropriate to give the floor to British philosopher Bertrand Russell (1872-1970):

> *Contempt for happiness is usually contempt for other people's happiness, and is an elegant disguise for hatred of the human race.*
> – from: *Portraits From Memory & Other Essays* (1956)

Given the lack of a cast iron guarantee about God's existence, the preservation of the soul after death or the meaning of life – not to mention the innate subjectivity, self-serving bias and obvious sensory and temporal limitations of human perception and thinking – we are at liberty to insert happiness into the gap when considering what our reasons might be for adopting certain beliefs. After all, what's wrong with happiness?

So, back to the question floated a few paragraphs ago – are we happy believing what we're believing? Are these beliefs helping us to live the life we would rather or are they, in fact, getting in the way and laying traps for us? Do our beliefs punish us? Force us? Make us stick with jobs that bore us shitless and prompt us to buy all sorts of crap we neither need nor genuinely want?

Of course, the answers here will be mixed – some yes, some no and plenty of possibly – because this is life, not some infantile Disney plotline.

Thus, given that what we're left with is a whole lot of nuance, complexity and incomplete information, we can now safely abandon the quest for the one true answer that puts absolutely everything right in favour of a more graduated, cost/benefit approach that allows us an ideology free space to go forward based entirely on our own best judgement.

Once more, the economist's conceptual kitbag will come in handy, because it allows for various and competing inputs and makes room for inconsistency and uncertainty. Remember the Potential Happiness Index (PHI) we explored in Chapter 2?

$$PH = \frac{\frac{\left(\frac{C}{T}\right) + A + Eq}{\left(\frac{V}{R}\right) + \left(\frac{O}{E}\right)} + W}{T}$$

PH = Potential Happiness
C = Capacity (overall health)
T = Time remaining (estimated in years)
A = Sense of Achievement
Eq = Equanimity (sense of calm & balance)
V = Validation (need for)
R = Relationships (importance of)
O = Obligations (importance of)
E = Ethics (importance of)
W = Wherewithal (finance, networks, conditions)

Flaky maths aside, the idea behind the PHI is to acknowledge the impact of and allow us to disentangle the relationship between the numerous factors that feed into our most important life choices – and in doing so to get a picture of how our perceptions about ourselves, others and the world affect our potential for happiness. Whilst happiness may well be a journey rather than a destination, the intention behind the PHI is to throw some focus onto the vehicle we're travelling in.

So, to better illustrate the potential impact of habitual, socially received beliefs and the power of slave narratives, let's get creative.

Meet Jan, a 34 year old IT consultant – male or female depending on your preferred pronunciation. Although well-educated and comfortably upper-middle class, Jan is convinced that an Orwellian, uber-nanny state is being engineered by a cadre of imperialist patriarchs, whilst simultaneously believing that everything unfolds as it should. Destiny notwithstanding, Jan strives relentlessly to be happy, wealthy and wise and to bring about justice for animals and better incomes for Asian textile workers. This, Jan believes, is what s/he came here for; it's part of their divine higher purpose and the next stage of their soul's journey towards nirvana. And yet, Jan is also relentlessly groovy, constantly waxing off extraneous body hair, seeking out the coolest dance tunes and telling all 4231 of their Facebook friends about every micro-bar, Tantric sex workshop and protest march they appear at. (In fact, anything less than 200 Likes per post usually results in a crippling bout of 'nobody loves me' gloom and self-doubt.)

One day Jan bumps into another former employee of the Evil Sludge Corporation – our recently divorced cancer suffering chum, Bourgeois Buddhist from Chapter 2 – who simply cannot wait to show their younger companion the PHI app on their latest 'augmented reality' iThing. Although pretending to be coolly unimpressed, the moment Jan gets home s/he jumps online and types in some numbers.

	SCORE	NOTE
Capacity	90%	Gym and yoga, healthy diet, regime of vitamin supplements, etc
Time remaining	50 years	Healthy choices will extend life, destiny notwithstanding
Achievement	3.5	Still so much to achieve
Equanimity	4.5	Still restless to achieve, fighting the world, etc
Validation	9	Is tempted to put less but has to confess
Relationships	8	Family, community, friends – a vital support network, etc
Obligations	8	Sense of duty driven by family, relationships and life purpose

	SCORE	**NOTE**
Ethics	9	Social and eco consciousness drives them
Wherewithal *	3.625	* as a result of $W = En(F+N)$
Environment	25%	Dystopian future, chem trails, micro-chipping people, etc
Finances	9	Not poor but would love to travel more, own a better house, etc
Networks	8	That community thing again, all those Facebook friends

PHI	**0.170**

Feeding Jan's figures into the equation and calculating to three decimal places we arrive at a potential happiness index of 0.170, which translates as a mere 17%.

This does not compare well with the scenarios we imagined in Chapter 2, those involving our fictional CEO and the aforementioned Bourgeois Buddhist. Even their lowest scores – 35.2% and 44.7% respectively – far exceed Jan's.

True, I have deliberately amplified Jan's proclivities, but my guess is that you probably know people like this – in the mirror or elsewhere. Their overarching sense of duty, their validation addiction, their 'victim's eye' view of the world and their constant struggle to be better, cooler and more enlightened adds up to a whole mountain of should, should, should. In risk/reward terms Jan's portfolio of beliefs seems to me like a very poor investment.

Beliefs which translate as command, or which have the effect of continuously whipping you or tethering you to the obligations legislated by customs, families or deities – or which mire you in a state of pre-apocalyptic dread and/or generate a sense of missing out, not being good enough or always wanting more – are simply not worth sticking with.

Seems like now is as good a time as any to sell out of that position.

THE MINIMAL BELIEF STRATEGY

Once we learn to apply the utility blowtorch to our beliefs – and to divest those which don't contribute positively to our potential for ongoing happiness – we are soon prompted to ask another question: why believe anything at all?

Far from being a petulant or merely poetic protest, this question merits serious attention – not least because it underlines once again that beliefs are principally voluntary. However, the real value in asking this is realised when we begin to accept that we can be genuinely certain of a very few and tightly limited range of things; and so therefore it behoves us not to be too dogmatic and locked into position.

To use the investor metaphor yet again – why park all your capital in a tight range of stocks? As you are probably aware, savvy investors looking for sustainable long-term returns almost always take a diversified portfolio, spreading their risk across the market. It is, after all, a smart move to acknowledge that incomplete information and personal bias, along with volatile and uncertain market movements, will mean that any portfolio is likely to contain a mix of profit and loss-making stocks. Really, it's basic 'eggs in basket' stuff. After all, there is no such thing as a guarantee in the market and *every* investment is a risk.

So too it is with what we tell ourselves about the world and our place within it. Hard ideological investment in this ism or that ology is a high risk, ultimately unsustainable position. What's more, painting yourself too firmly into a dogmatic corner will come at the cost of flexibility, adaptability and openness to new opportunity.

Or, to defer to Bertrand Russell again:

> *The whole problem with the world is that fools and fanatics are always so certain of themselves, and wiser people so full of doubts.*
> – from: *The Triumph Of Stupidity* (1933)

> *I would never die for my beliefs because I might be wrong.*
> – from: Leonard Lyons in the *New York Post* (1964) – quoting a conversation he had with Russell

Whilst the imprimatur of Mr Russell is in itself no guarantee of correctness, it has been the experience and observation of many that 'certainty' equates not simply with arrogance and intransigence but can also play out in unnecessary suffering for the self and the cruel treatment of others. Do Wahhabist suicide bombers thoughtfully weigh up shades of grey on their way to exterminate women and children in marketplaces? *Hey look, maybe there really aren't any gorgeously fuckable virgin babes on tap up there in Heaven but hey, why don't we just blow ourselves up on the off chance?*

The obvious point here is not to believe too strongly in too much – but in my experience the real joy of the 'doubt default' goes beyond the mere equivocation of existential hedging, or betting both ways. Indeed, it makes space for a kind of lightness. For whatever else they are, beliefs are also baggage. Yet, once we can surrender the idea that we have to work everything out, that the right belief will lead us to some kind of jackpot, we realise that to a large extent it simply does not matter what we believe – by which I mean, even my belief in not believing won't prevent me being murdered by IS operatives, eaten by a shark or sexually rejected by the next person I become entranced by.

In fact, to be blunt, in the main, belief is a waste of time. Sure, very useful at certain times – like when we believe that avoiding cars when crossing roads is a good thing – but when it comes to gods, grand encompassing narratives and the idea that a bigger house will result in a happier life, it's a very ill-advised gamble indeed.

Meanwhile, the rewards of non-belief can be measured in reduced stress, a sense of personal liberty and empowerment, and a whole bunch of mental and emotional energy freed up for more joyful pursuits than building up and defending a citadel of faith.

In my personal experience, there was a very rewarding symbiosis between unshackling myself from formerly cherished notions and a general ability to just let shit go. What's more, once I learned to regard my beliefs as simply habits, patterned responses, I was able to arrest the previously 'inevitable' momentum of my thoughts, feelings and behaviours earlier in the loop, and therefore present myself with opportunities for conscious choice.

Would I like to continue down this well-worn path or … ?

As simple and banal as this sounds, my topical conscious awareness of this – in the moment – creates a freedom of choice that so many of my companions in the highly privileged West tell themselves they don't have. And sure, it's not a silver bullet or quick fix, but it continues to be a very effective means of focusing my attention and giving me the opportunity to execute change and shift my existential market position around to create better yields.

Drilling down a little further, the more rigid a portfolio of beliefs the less likely the believer is to genuinely act in the moment, according to the situation at hand, and the more likely they are to apply pre-packaged solutions and resort to familiar and often unconscious response patterns. I'm sure I don't need to outline exactly why *that* is a dumb strategy.

But suffice it to say, eradicating *all* belief would also be a bad call (aside, that is, from being practically impossible for social primates living in highly ordered societies; or indeed Earth bound animals making assumptions about gravity and so on). For instance, when I eat breakfast I do so in the belief that, most likely, later in the day I will also get to eat lunch, dinner, etc. I don't know *absolutely* that civilisation won't collapse at 11:36am, thus derailing my plans for a light midday snack, or that I won't abruptly die at 2:12pm, but I behave as if I do. Clearly, on a risk/reward basis, it pays for me to eat breakfast in a relaxed and relatively confident fashion (there will be other breakfasts) as opposed to scoffing down a meal that I think may well be my last. And sure, whilst the condemned prisoner's last meal may indeed be an almost religious experience of pure taste, I'm personally inclined to take the slightly less delicious breakfast option over the idea that I'll never have bacon & eggs again.

I mention this; a) to idiot/pedant proof my basic contention about not believing too much, and; b) to point again at the pragmatic clarity that can be gained from utilising the cost/benefit prism and the economic metaphor more generally. Any belief system – even a minimalist one – has downside risk. The perfect portfolio is not possible in a dynamic world, but a prudent and practised risk metrics mechanism opens up a window of opportunity to assess how best to invest our most precious assets – time, passion, etc.

To conclude – given that I know I don't know everything and that some things are most likely impossible for an ephemeral, self-identifying consciousness complex to ever know – my response to the uncertainty is to accept that, since my beliefs will often tend toward self-serving assertion, they might as well *really* serve me. As in:

- Allow me a sense of self-authoring.
- Underpin operating assumptions about sanity, competence and self-worth.
- Engender the psychological conditions and behavioural traits most likely to deliver sustainable happiness.

For me at any rate, this is the brief when it comes to belief.

8.
THE PEOPLE'S REPUBLIC OF POINTLESSNESS

or

Your completely meaningless lifestyle guide

At its core, meaning is a survival tool – it's about navigating the uncertain terrain of life. It is a useful if incomplete map, a bunch of clues about where we are and where we wish to go. It is our existential lighthouse. So let's just hope it's not luring us onto the rocks.

In this chapter I appraise common notions of meaning and confront the phenomenon of 'spiritual correctness' before investigating the risks and rewards of the pointless p.o.v. and the art of living lightly.

So far in this book we have teased out a number of inter-related psychological and philosophical strands and used metaphors and conceptual frameworks drawn from economics to address questions concerning happiness; or how we might find ways to live the life we want as opposed to one we feel compelled to. Along the way we have focused on a few key themes:

- Fear of death and the denialist culture of command and control it has spawned.
- The imprisoning power of narratives – political and spiritual ideologies, social and moral dogmas, etc.
- Attainment mania – socially visible status, corporate ladders, musts and bucket lists, etc.
- Freedom, responsibility and the easy lure of slave narratives.
- The power of our beliefs to either liberate or subjugate us.

However, rather than insisting on a new orthodoxy or imposing yet another straightjacket of 'permanence' on you, I have argued for a more fluid mode of negotiating the uncertainties and unknowables of life. To this end I have called upon the much maligned discipline of economics, co-opting ideas around the assigning and weighting of perceived value and the analysis of risk versus reward (or cost/benefit). In doing this I have not only suggested that time is our most valuable asset but endeavoured to create a starting point model (the PHI) for examining how the ways we value and prioritise things can either enhance or adversely impact our potential for present and future happiness.

Running through all this is a pretty simple idea that in a constantly changing and evolving world it seems prudent for us to mirror the fundamental symbiotic dynamism of existence in the structure of our beliefs and practises – indeed, to understand and accept that we are not *external* to this world. That, in fact, everything about us, including everything we think and feel, takes place entirely *within* the continuously morphing, flexible world (nature, reality, etc) we find ourselves in.

Which brings us now to the titular point; namely, pointlessness.

Previously, I have elaborated the idea that freeing ourselves from the fascism of meaning, from the reductionist rigidity of 'about' and 'here for' is one of the keys to a profound and life-altering liberation. In this chapter, I will expand upon this and, in doing so, try to sow the seeds of a revolution. Because the time is right for a little spiritual sedition.

THE MEANING OF MEANING

Before we get into the so-called meaning of life, I'd like to take a little detour and ponder what we *mean* by meaning. What is a purpose, what is a point, etc – and how do they arise? Sure, this is normally one for the teleology nerds out there, (like the word *teleology* itself, which refers to the purpose of stuff), but it's also useful and illustrative for the rest of us to drill into these things, if only to expose complacent assumptions and open up new avenues of possibility.

Let's start with language, where meaning comes about through consensus (we all agree that a certain sound signifies a certain object, common experience, action, etc) but also through context. For instance, every word in this sentence exists in a 'relationship of meaning' with every other word. Indeed, in its day to day use, language is a social technology, a group code, and is therefore rooted in our relationship with each other and the world more broadly. In addition to its role as the namer and describer of the world (objects, phenomena, qualities, intentions, etc) it also serves as a tool for condensing our vaguer desires and more abstract ideas into a communicable form. Language lets us indicate what we mean in addition to creating entirely new categories and intricacies of meaning. In a way, words are the quanta of meaning.

But of course, this strictly semantic kind of meaning is not what we are referring to when we ask what does life mean? However, even when we *do* speak of meaning in this more existential/metaphysical space, 'relationship' still lies at the core of it. Why? Because meanings (or purposes, or points) cannot exist in isolation. In a world of just one. Neither can they exist in steady states – in other words, *outside* of fluid, networked, temporal universes. For just as we cannot talk about information without also implying transmission – signals sent *and* received – the notion of meaning makes no sense in a universe where nothing happens or where there is no differentiation between x and not x, and where the x and the not x don't interact. Thus, meaning requires both time (flux) and context (relationship) in order to arise.

And of course all this higher meaning and purpose stuff, all these grand overarching points, cannot occur without a minimum level of awareness. Without an atomised perspective or particularity.

Existence includes the I

Whatever your opinion of the I – ego, self, etc – the fact is that the event of your encapsulated, self-identifying human consciousness (or life) happens as *part* of the unfolding, interwoven, dynamic flow of the universe. Every single aspect of your living is *included* in the overall existence complex. Obvious though this may seem, humanity has long been in the habit of regarding itself as an outside observer. Partly, this is an understandable side effect of I/Not I; yet it is also, paradoxically, a false dichotomy. For just as we are not separate from what we call nature, our experience as an incrementally developing, consistent narrative of becoming (and ultimately unbecoming) not only parallels the structure and flux of the cosmos but is simply one of its vast array of emergent phenomena. Thus, human conscious identity is an enigmatic duality – a process that 'sees' itself to such an extent that it can self-edit on the fly. Life is a self-correcting mechanism. Identity is homeostatic.

Bringing this down from the metaphysical stratosphere, we might interpret this as an existential invitation to 'make it up as you go along', to gaze into the mirror of being and enter into a life-long, co-dependent relationship with yourself. Or simply to know thyself – and by the very act of knowing make real. In this context, pass/fail judgements and either/or meaning tropes are surely an utter irrelevance.

So, quite aside from whether you think flowers, fish or whole universes have life meanings and conscious long term objectives, or whether indeed you believe they simply follow procedure, (obeying mathematical laws, adapting or dying out, or even pursuing what Aristotle call 'telos'), it is clear that the locus of meaning is specific viewpoint. The life purpose of a bee, such as it is, exists entirely within the context of bee-ness; even if the bee's purpose also supports the telos of pollen and birds and the honey eating proclivities of certain bipedal primates. Thus, as a human being, or iterated identity complex (ego, self, etc) able to consistently distinguish between the I and the Not I – in essence, as someone who exists *in a world* and experiences *a life* – you are the generator and selector of a meaning portfolio tailored to reflect your human-ness and serve your anthropogenic intentions. Furthermore, it is only through the act of relating with the world that all your notions of meaning become possible and are derived; and although the world profoundly influences not only your choices but who you think you are, in the end it's *you* who gets to say what, if anything, the point is. Even if you're just agreeing with the mullah or bumbling along with the destiny puppets.

If I was of the Essentialist persuasion though, I might say something like: so if the universe *is* consciousness doesn't that imply the possibility that the universe has some kind of alpha-objective, primary meaning or telos? Or that meaning is innate. Ordained externally. Pre-authorised. Part of the very fabric and function of existence.

This is an entirely valid question. However, it's a bit like asking what the point of existence is. Why, as some philosophers muse, is there something rather than nothing? Why would a God, a supposedly perfect one at that, create anything at all? To simply state, as New Agers and quantum mysticists are wont to, that the universe (God, cosmic consciousness, et al) wants to know it, him or herself serves only to generate further questions.

- Is there an underlying reason, other than to exist, that the universe wants to know itself?
- In fact, can we really say that the universe 'wants' to know itself rather than just knowing itself because that's what the universe, or existence, *is* – namely, the very act of self-knowing, of self-becoming?
- And once the universal self is known why would this necessarily imply any subsequent objectives – moral, spiritual, historical or otherwise?
- Indeed, why or how would this vast cosmic act of self-knowing be in any way reduced to aspirational or ideological imperative – wouldn't it just include every single thing within the ambit of becoming itself, rather than limiting itself to prescribed linear/narrative purposes?

All of which brings us back to relationship. If we really want to say that the universe (existence) has a purpose other than simply the self-contained intention to *be* – or indeed that the great cosmic mirror gazing routine occurred as a result of a prior intention to know the self – we are positing a locus of meaning *external* to existence. From there it's just infinite regress, tautology and admittedly entertaining paradoxes. Great for symposiums and late night stoner sessions but not necessarily salient for answering questions about how to live a more genuinely fulfilling life.

The other thing that leaps out here is that our various conceptualisations of meaning are almost invariably related to notions of function and problem solving. Life meaning theories are a response to philosophical and existential conundrums like the ones listed above, and nearly all of them attempt, in some way, to address the question of how to live the best life possible. Everything from following God's moral curriculum, to the more survivalist/evolutionary 'error correction for fitness' models, ground life purpose in a good/bad, pass/fail framework that binds the nominated ends to a set of means. We can *achieve* our goals, *realise* our Heavenly intended purpose, *lift* our vibration – and all via the agency of proper function. Best practise. Whether that's evolving to sync better with environmental changes or simply following divine instruction.

From here it is no wonder that, as they map out into our everyday lives and are enunciated by mere mortals, most life meaning tropes soon lurch into moralising, controlling, reductionist, tick box, either/or mantras underwritten by fear, vanity, blame shifting and anthropomorphisation. Indeed, our ideas around meaning in the 'whole of life' context more often than not manifest as a kind of comfort pillow or safe space – a narrative palliative, neatly simplifying a complex and uncontrollable world and soothing our existential terrors; with punishment mechanisms frequently on hand to help keep us in line.

At its core, meaning is a survival tool – it's about navigating the uncertain terrain of life. It is a useful if incomplete map, a bunch of clues about where we are and where we wish to go. It is our existential lighthouse. So let's just hope it's not luring us onto the rocks.

I ♥ ENLIGHTENMENT CHIC

As noted in previous chapters, in the post-WW2 West the enlightenment craze has resulted not only in the fashionable adoption of Eastern and First Nation philosophies and cosmologies but in the pop culture cherry picking of theoretical physics. Beginning with writers like Alan Watts and Beat Generation 'dharma bums' like Jack Kerouac, the vogue for spiritual alternatives to Christianity, capitalism and materialism soon moved from intellectual and literary bohemia to undergrad hippiedom and thence through the New Age to the solipsism and outright hubris of the middle class 'manifestation' cult. Indeed, I don't think it's too unkind to suggest that a majority of our bourgeois bodhisattva friends have concocted a version of higher truth designed to legitimise their own selfishness and bathe them in the warm glow of a supposedly alt-wisdom.

However, much as we might deride the commodification of enlightenment as little more than Disney dharma – a kind of 'me, me, me in designer kaftans' with a happy ending and a thousand Likes on Facebook – there remains something undeniably genuine about it. For sitting beneath the numerous poses and obvious hypocrisies is a desire for meaning. Boiled down, the core question is typically: why am I here? This then fans out into things like:

- Is there a purpose to life beyond reproduction – am I here for a pre-ordained, non-genetic reason?
- Is there something I am supposed to do, learn or discover?

- Is there a super-purpose for humanity – have we evolved this way to achieve a certain objective?
- Is my life a kind of prep school or entrance exam for a post-death existence – a step on a ladder, turn of a wheel, ticket to heaven or hell?
- Is there something more than eat/shit, sleep/wake, work/consume, fuck/die?
- Does all, or indeed any of this, actually fucking mean something – and if so, what?

These are age old musings and our species has endeavoured to address them in a number of ways – animist, theist, pan-psychist, scientific and so on. The currently chic and sexily self-improved enlightenment consumers are simply the latest, probably richest, maybe fattest pilgrims to tread the path and visit the mega-mall of meaning – credit cards at the ready. And of course, they are not the first to litter the road to nirvana with self-serving delusion, denial, arrogance, righteous judgement and petty control narratives.

Partly because we have culturally and individually put so much time and energy into seeking and finding enlightenment we have, as a corollary, also made it into a cynosure of our desire. It has become a life objective. The quest to uncover true meaning *is* a meaning in and of itself. Along the way, enlightenment has also proved to be a useful tool of division, of sifting out the good from the not so good, the saints from the sinners and the awakened from the sheeple. This brand of so-called wisdom is a shiny fetish object, a socially visible marker of achievement and worthiness. A trophy for the self-anointed holy champions. A tick for the spiritually correct.

Subsequently, we tell ourselves that because these teleological superstars have gained superior insight they must surely have stumbled across the keys to a more meaningful existence. *Fuck, they know what they're here for, don't they? They're not randomly blundering around doing shit jobs or crying over spilt milk, are they? I mean, they* are *living a better life, right?*

Right?

I mean, that's what it's for, isn't it? That's what meaning is meant to deliver – a better, more fulfilling, less fearful, less confusing, happier overall life? Otherwise, what's the fucking point of there being a point to everything? In fact, if the upshot of working out the ultimate reason for life, the universe and everything is simply to confirm me as an accountability dodging slave, unredeemable sinner/victim or anaesthetised time server – a cog in a deterministic machine or an intrinsically unworthy speck of crud crawling the cosmic sidewalk for a shot of spiritual smack – enlightenment be damned. Unless of course …

GETTING OVER SPIRITUAL CORRECTNESS

What if there was nothing to work out? Or what if you just accepted that, even if there *was* some grand, unifying point to everything, you were never going to know it? Suppose you said to yourself:

What are the chances that something as amazingly complex as an entire universe – or as paradoxically mysterious as existence – would align itself to the pettiness and vanity of ego-driven purpose or the childlike neatness of storybook narrative?

Taking that thought further, you might soon wonder: what are the chances that the entirety of existence somehow resembles a person, or indeed possesses narrowly defined, human values or perspectives? Why, you might ask, would a universe need to mean anything at all? And what possible purpose could there be for something as all-inclusive as existence? With what could 'the everything' enter into a relationship of meaning with? What (and indeed when and where) is the context that would allow possible 'meanings of everything' to arise?

Although the two most common answers to this question, as already noted, are God and 'itself', neither of these *necessarily* imply linear meaning, nor indeed any kind of ethical or attainment based system. Therefore, given that none of us can reasonably claim 100% certainty in this regard, it wouldn't be out of the ballpark for us to nominate odds in the region of several centrillion* to one for the notion that existence somehow legislates a central, over-riding point to our lives and that this uber-meaning coincidentally mirrors the perspectives and objectives of one species on one planet in the outer arm of one of several billion galaxies. In which case you may as well give up trying to second guess the cosmos and just decide for yourself what your life means. I mean, pick your battles, folks.
(* 10^{303} in the short scale, or 10^{600} in the long scale.)

Having got this far, suppose you then just abandoned the whole idea of alpha-meaning or super-purpose altogether? What if you could forget the grand plan completely? Maybe, instead of having a single, defining point you could have several points; and perhaps, instead of them being rigid and reductionist (mission based or underpinned by pass/fail criteria), these multiple points could be vaguer, more flexible guidelines or aspirations.

Okay, so there's the nagging fear of being wrong (straying off track, going down a blind alley, risking the wrath of a pissed off God) and the parallel dread of missing out on the reputedly golden and eternal rewards of rightness – but what if the schoolroom right/wrong dichotomy became an irrelevance? After all, if we step back far enough, things that seem crucial up close eventually retract into insignificance. From the 'whole of existence' perspective it's difficult to figure out how the minutiae of human affairs would be particularly important, or even register as anything more than a blip-sized fraction of the blipiest blip you could ever imagine.

Indeed, even if you take the view that you are the *whole ocean in a drop*, as opposed to a drop *in* an ocean, your 'whole of ocean-ness' precludes, by definition, any possibility of meta-oceanic authority to mark you right or wrong or set tasks for you. At either end of the scale – infinitesimally tiny ape or cosmic sized hyper-consciousness – you are left to your own devices. Either the universe doesn't particularly notice or care that much about you, or you *are* the universe and therefore not bound by anyone else's rules or plans for you since, y'know, there is nobody but you.

Oh and another thing – if you're really genuine about your beliefs in this space and they're not just pretty, clever sounding things to spout at dinner parties or post as memes, in both models you are stripped of the handy higher authority get out clause so beloved of slave-thinkers everywhere.

My intention in all this isn't merely to kill off Gods or cast you into an uncaring void but to illustrate the ways in which the stories we tell ourselves about higher meaning and ultimate purpose shackle us by keeping us in a childlike dependence/resentment relationship with the parental/external. And what's more, if all we do by way of response is replace the countless external voices of judgement and control with an internal disciplinarian of our own concoction, we are still imprisoning ourselves in a tunnel of pre-determined spiritual correctness. Replacing the punishments of others with the scoldings of the self is, in my estimation, a disastrously bad investment of your energy and time.

Because, let's remind ourselves why we're here – me typing, you reading. It's not about revealing the best kept secrets of existence or parading our wisdom for the genuflection and sexual favours of whoever we're into right now; it's about how to increase the likelihood of being happy going forward. How to more prudently invest our remaining time in things we like rather than stuff we're told we have to.

Naturally, our profundity wielding STW friends (those blessed Spiritual Truth Warriors determined to get us all vibrating in tune with their ideological frequency) will baulk at this. *Empty Nihilism*, they will decry. They may even castigate us for being lazy. *Ah, you're just copping out. This pointlessness shtick is nothing more than code for not bothering.*

True, on the face of it this book does indeed argue the case for not giving a fuck about much. Or, to put it more politely, detachment. Yes, I *am* suggesting that if we stop putting our focus and care into socially defined ideas about who we're meant to be and what we're all supposed to achieve, we can and probably will:

- Experience much less stress.
- More easily step back from wasteful competitive squabbles.
- Lay off the endless boasting and posing routines.
- Abandon our futile attempts to control stuff we can't and focus instead on putting our efforts into what we *can* influence – namely, our own thoughts and feelings about ourselves and the world and, by extension, the decisions we make and the actions we take.

Okay, I confess, it's not a recipe for nirvana or cosmos shattering insight but it *is* a pathway to freedom.

Furthermore, the *Pointless Revolution* is about existential courage. It's about taking responsibility and accepting uncertainty with equanimity; without recourse to puerile control mechanisms, the fantasy of bedtime story encapsulations, or the 24/7 convenience of other blaming. It's about having the guts to stop being a slave and to create and allow yourself the scope to move however you chose. To change course, experiment, make mistakes, quit jobs, give the finger to tyrants and abusers, enjoy the sunshine, write novels, watch football, ignore fashion, get off treadmills and, crucially, not be afraid of death. None of that sounds especially like copping out to me.

Ultimately, to abandon the safety net of meaning is to be open to uncertainty and change, is to live more in the present and much less in an abstract, gotta do future. Just as overcoming the fear of death allows you to truly live, so dissolving the directives of divine higher purpose and tearing up the bucket list leaves you free to choose what *really* makes you happy – and then change your mind and do something else entirely.

Here again, the spiritual correctness police would most likely intervene. As I touched upon in the previous chapter, there exists a certain snootiness about mere happiness; as if somehow this is not a worthy enough goal. Heaven forfend that we should *enjoy* our lives. Whilst we might expect this kind of attitude from conservative Christians mired in a miserablist world of original sin and ideological self-loathing, I can also report raised eyebrows and mild scoffing from most of the people I've mentioned the writing of this book to. *Eew, happy*, they object, *isn't that a tad trivial? Surely there's something deeper than that to exercise your mind, Paulie.*

Um, okay, what exactly would that be then? Or are we simply getting bogged down in semantics? Perhaps we would prefer nice, educated middle class words like wisdom or clarity?

Unfortunately, pretty well all of us have been steeped so thoroughly in the prevailing spiritual culture – which is rooted in central denial and derides our experience as either sinful, a vale of illusion or a form of exam we are almost certain to abjectly fail – that we have come to view happiness as either wanton, perverse and unnatural, or as a sign of howling stupidity and/or profligacy. Or, if you think that's a tad overstated, that being happy is generally considered a lesser spiritual objective than higher learning or the pursuit of apparently meaningful life paths. *Happiness is for the poor little dummies down there. Up here, our truths are* much *higher.*

Step back from all this and what you observe is little more than a mode of control. So much of human spiritual tradition is predicated on judging you, comparing you to arbitrary external standards, telling you you're wrong about pretty well everything that matters, and getting you to sign up to orthodoxies that someone else invented.

In my view, the fiction of the uber-meaning is designed to co-opt us into a sphere of external control. The manifold strictures of enlightenment didacts operate both socially and personally, either by welcoming us to one of the various churchy bosoms or having us impose reductionist linear imperatives on ourselves. This is not to suggest that all existential inquiries and metaphysical musings are thought policing in disguise but rather to acknowledge the ingrained human social habit of imposing forms of spiritual correctness and conflating acquiescence with wisdom, morality and worthiness.

At this juncture, and in the spirit of the book, it seems appropriate to ask: why the fuck would you bother going along with any of that?

THE POINTLESS P.O.V.

As previously observed, (in Chapters 3-5), a full and grateful acceptance of mortality and a move away from the delusions of mattering are very much part of our *Pointless Revolution*. To most people this will seem counter-intuitive at best, downright negative and self-limiting at worst. Some will even say that to dispense with meaning is to push gateway drugs to suicide and cruelty. Though we have dealt with these objections earlier it is worth simply reminding these jittery folk that our shared human history is replete with cruelty, violence, oppression, megalomania, utterly myopic selfishness and other complacencies; much of which have been informed and underwritten by powerful meaning tropes and their attendant ideological imperatives. (Extremist Sunni Islam being one of the more lurid and spectacular new millennium examples.)

It is also prudent to remind ourselves once more that 'the pointless p.o.v.' is no guard against immorality and no marker of superiority. Indeed, when we throw off the yoke of meaning we are given only opportunity – the space to make choices and the potential to do whatever we want. It is an invitation to participate in a free market of life options, with a bunch of discretionary temporal capital to invest. It is *not* a stairway to heaven or a badge of honour.

Clearly, the abandoning of socially ordained meanings and the overthrowing of the parental/external authority complex does not come without risk. (Nothing does.) However, the key to making it stick and to increasing your potential for happiness is attitudinal. True, the world will throw curve balls at you – uncertainty is a given – but the flexibility allowed and the equanimity engendered by pointlessness makes it far more likely that you will be able to go with whatever flow is on; not as the grumbling victim of an overwhelming force but with gratitude and a sense of empowering perspective.

It's a big claim, I know – but here's why I think it's reasonable. Firstly, direct personal experience. I have lately learnt to put 'the pointless p.o.v.' into daily practise and am happy to report that it is working better and delivering healthier dividends than any alternative belief portfolio I may have employed in the past. Regular pay-offs in the form of a more broadly based general contentment, greater balance, more moments of sheer joy and a far greater ability to be in the present are just the headline benefits of this strategy*. Yet, beyond mere assertion, the space created by the metaphysical tabula rasa of pointlessness is a place that not only seems to invite but is *sustained* by gratitude – and in turn this thankfulness and ability to appreciate what you have, rather than fixating on what you *wish* you had, makes the supposedly mystical jackpot of being in the moment much more achievable. (* More of this in Appendix 3.)

Think of it like this:

- Life meanings, super-purposes, bucket lists, must imperatives, et al, focus your attention and desire on relatively fixed but abstract future points – in other words, future rewards for correct action/behaviour – be good, get sweets – enlighten well, get holy trophies.

- Depending on the strength with which you attend and adhere to your meaning beliefs, your attention and desire is necessarily funnelled – because now you are striding purposively towards something – you are more outcome focused – you walk a path.

- Once you clearly define that path you automatically co-define the antonymous idea of deviation – of being wrong, fucking it up, missing out, not collecting enough experiences, going to hell, being a loser.

- As a side effect you have now set up a pass/fail dichotomy that fuels self-punishment and punitive judgement, not to mention a mechanism that allows you to pre-judge and crudely essentialise others – as well as honing the cutting edge of the judgements that others foist upon you and potentially informing a distorting sense of your own entitlement.

And so therefore:

- In contrast, having no clearly defined meaning and/or enlightenment directive defuses the power of the imagined (abstract) future point and allows your attention and desire to come back more into the (concrete) now – effectively altering your risk/reward position by freeing you up to take a bigger punt on finding joy in the present.

- Furthermore, without the ideological overhang of right/wrong, good/bad, either/or you can operate from a more fearless and potentially punishment free position – because now you can't possibly fail at life – your mistakes are only mistakes, not grievous sins or karmic downgrades – the universe won't be offended by your trenchant recalcitrance – your 'experience collection' won't ever be star rated by tattooed fifteen year old hipsters in skinny jeans.

- Also, having weaned yourself off the 'whole point of everything' drug, the opium of narrative ceases to be so addictive and you find yourself much less attracted to the knee blanket of simplistic, catch-all explanations; and thus you put less effort into the wasteful and potentially damaging pursuit of the ultimate truth(s) and, as an additional benefit, you also shed the multiple conceits of the wisdom seeker – which in turn serves to allow your focus to drift back from future solutions and heavenly rewards to a more grateful present.

- The really huge pay-off in 'present focus' is not so much spiritual as psycho-emotional and practical – the now pays out right now, with dividends in joy, reduced stress, less punishment and the kind of 'grateful for what is right in front of me' attitude that renders sustainable long term happiness and freedom much more likely.

Suffice it to say that a belief portfolio based more on and/also and less upon hardwired either/or distinctions also in-builds a level of adaptability; a latitude not constricted by pre-arranged ideological objectives or by the fear of not attaining them. Weave a good measure of gratitude into the mix and suddenly you are no longer operating out of lack and dread because you are more able to extract value from what you already have. Those incessant more, more, more mantras just stop being convincing.

And of course, the 'have to' lie is fully revealed. Without mandated end points and the vindictive, judgemental, bullying numina required to enforce their spiritual law, there is no compulsion. No must finish, must arrive, must tick off that goddam list. The classics of slavespeak – I should, I'm being forced to, etc – are replaced by I can, I will, I'd really like to and so on.

Blend this with a more fearless attitude to death and you soon begin to understand that even being alive is a choice. In fact, it's that very decision – to stay living – which, when rescued from habit, dread and genetic impulse, and brought out into the conscious light, can fuel a profound yet pragmatic shift in attitude and, as a result, support the momentum for *actual* change in your life. Y'know, change you can believe in. ☺

Emoticons notwithstanding, I do not say this lightly. Indeed, properly examined, I believe that this realisation can kickstart a massively liberating and empowering process of re-appraising our core life choices and the often unchallenged beliefs that underpin them. For a start, there is a big difference between 'I'm hanging on because I'm petrified of death' and 'I choose to be alive because the sensation is so vital, extraordinary and beautiful.' What's more – and without wishing to sound glib, righteous or unduly repetitive – we are, in fact, all 100% free to end the private, angsty spectacle of our slavery and suffering whenever we choose. The woeful clichéd objections and moralising melodramas around suicide are just so much fear and self-pity in bemoaning hypocritical disguise. If society's best argument against suicide amounts to little more than emotional blackmail and platitude it's not exactly a ringing endorsement of life. Likewise, the spiritually correct (with their judgmental Gods, divine 'to do' lists and destiny directives) see fit to offer only compulsion, punishment, servitude and a side dish of vanity as reasons to keep living. However, once we learn to ignore the voices of command and control, and accept that we remain alive because we *choose to be* then we underscore in bold existential terms the fundamental core upon which our freedom is founded.

Because, if you can choose to die, you can choose to live – and actively *choosing* to live is not the same as just staying alive, as not wanting to die.

To some this may seem banal, if not trivial and facetious, but it goes to the heart of the central denial and deflates the mythologies it supports. For as long as we defer to a *reason* for being alive, we are effectively saying that we're only here because we have to be. Even if we elevate evolution or brute materialist determinism to the function of 'ultimate point' we are establishing an external mechanism of validating, legitimising authority and reducing the phenomenon of life to the pursuit of pre-determined objectives or the execution of cosmic choreography.

JUST BECAUSE

And so the question is asked: what *is* the bloody point then?

But again that's just the point; there isn't one, and neither do we need to make one up. Surely we're over that tired old point business by now?

That said, we'd be dishonest if we tried to deny that we didn't crave at least *some* form of meaning in our lives. Some framework of guiding principles, however minimal. And perhaps too a self-serving sense of persistent underlying purpose; not only to help us maintain and bolster the notion of 'our character' but to make the bother of getting out of bed seem worthwhile. Or, to put it in economic terms, so that the benefits of living outweigh the costs and that the locked in sunset clause of death doesn't dampen our appetite for risk or make us easy prey for spiritual scammers and marketing sharks.

Thus, in lieu of the return on our existential market position being the absolute, final revealed truth and the attendant ecstasy of its revelation, I am of the view that the best available dividend payable between now and death is happiness – and that whatever beliefs we adopt and stories we tell ourselves about what our life is supposedly 'for', they should broadly deliver the goods. Even if they sometimes involve a little fiction. (For instance, I have my own sustaining self-mythology, principally around the kind of guy I am and the kind of life I think is worth living; and even if these narratives do sometimes stray from the hard literal truth or fail to align with what others would gladly tell you about me, as long as these stories don't result in harm to others and leave me free to reap a good flow of happiness dividends, I'll take them as a win.)

Reading this, you may well be thinking 'hang on a minute, haven't you just spent ages convincing us to give up on meaning?' Indeed yes; but note also that I have consistently argued that we are, all of us, the makers of private meaning. In effect what I have been outlining in this chapter particularly, and in the book generally, is that our commonly received, socially vetted ideas about life purpose are based on a didactic, authoritarian architecture rocket fuelled by mortal terror and the fear of exclusion – in addition to being heavily informed by denial and propped up by a serious lack of intellectual rigour. Therefore, in order to ameliorate the debilitating and enslaving effects of the ubiquitous parental/external authority complex and its infantile storybook simplicities, we need an edifice of meaning built on something other than fear.

What if there was a model of meaning that was not about performing certain functions in order to satisfy externally imposed criteria? What if it went a little further than dressed up approval seeking? Imagine if the meaning of your life had nothing whatsoever to do with the moral of someone else's story? Suppose you had nothing to prove?

The trick here is balance. Something like the famous middle path that Buddhists speak of. On one hand you want to liberate yourself from the service of reductionist, punishing ideology, whilst on the other you want to create a believable sense that you're doing something a little more enervating and inspiring than waiting in the queue for death. Effectively, you're looking to find the right mix of blunt truth and comforting fantasy; a pragmatist's suspension of disbelief that keeps you functioning happily without dragging you into denial, hubris and infantile fantasy.

For me, the best candidate in this space is obvious. It requires no gods, no moral or other tests of virtue, and it mandates no end goal or alpha narrative. Although it never tells me I'm bad because I did this or didn't that, or tries to convince me that *things* would be much better if only *I* was better – it *does* make me accountable for my actions or lack thereof. Whilst it is rich with nuance, ambiguity and uncertainty, it remains remarkably simple.

The bedrock reason I choose to stay alive, the core motivation for getting up, doing stuff, taking risks, enduring setbacks and all the rest of it is … well really, just because. I *choose* to live *for the sake of it*. For the sheer beauty of being a self that experiences *a life* in a world. I am no longer on a path, I am just walking. And while I walk I smell the flowers, taste the fruit, feel the brush of the air and – if you'll pardon the pun – see the light.

A process/outcome thing

During a recent catch-up with a friend she asked me how a certain (film) project was going and I mentioned that it was primarily dependent on whether or not the funding was approved. I said, "If the money happens then …" and she castigated me at once, insisting that I instead say, "*When* the money happens …" After making it clear that I did not share her belief in manifestation, she continued to argue that I was dooming myself to so-called failure with my "negative" wording. "On the contrary," I replied. "To say 'when' not only focuses on but *assumes* an outcome and, therefore, sows the seed of potential disappointment and perceived failure; whereas 'if' softens the focus on outcome, creates more room for gratitude and removes the fear associated with being let down." Still she insisted that I would "never succeed with that attitude" so I asked her what 'success' was. "Whereas your focus is on an external future outcome, mine is on a present feeling state," was my basic point. "To me, being happy this afternoon and not fretting about whether or not this film will ever happen *is* success."

Why do I mention this now? Because the 'process not outcome' thing that we're all familiar with is analogous to the 'pointless p.o.v.' I am suggesting in this chapter. Viewed through a risk/reward prism, making the process fun seems to me like a much better bet that fixating on either/or outcomes – just as living lightly and 'for the sake of it' strikes me as being a far superior way forward than shackling myself to pre-determined objectives and alpha-meanings, let alone to the petulant, wishful thinking, entitlement fantasies of manifestation.

From the limited, idiosyncratic perspective of the self-awareness event that I call 'me' I am *experiencing* both a self and a world in a symbiotic dance of such exquisitely patterned information exchange that it gives rise to the intoxicating riches of stuff like love and melancholy, art and ideas, the aroma of coffee and the shape of a woman. I may never know the truth but every single day I am free to find the fragile spectacle of living utterly beautiful.

In saying this I am not declaring special status or poetic nobility, nor staking any kind of claim to enlightenment. However, what I can say is that the 'for the sake of it' position generates a kind of lightness. Uncluttered by ideology, with no delusions or imperatives around rightness or particular mission, this is an existential investment strategy that sheds the weight of expectation, evaporates the pressure to succeed and compete, and seriously reduces the nagging desire for bigger, better, etc. In addition, it blows the cobwebs out of your head, making either/or largely irrelevant and allowing you to adopt more flexible and/also positions. And of course, it lets you tear up every single one of those karmic/cosmic moral exam papers. In fact, you can ditch that school altogether.

Living lightly, so to speak, also has the benefit of giving you the mental and emotional space to make critical decisions without the crushing burden of must. It also lets you deal with the various forms of despair without undue pathologisation, without regarding the hard times as either punishment, legislated samsara or as a sign of your intrinsic weakness or lack of worth.

Indeed, this approach lets you see everything that happens in your life – including your life – as simply an event; as opposed to being a point on a plotline intended to elucidate some arcane moral or vainglorious cosmic hero drama. Or, to put it another way, it lets you focus more easily on the present by snapping off the super-structures that keep your attention nailed to abstract future outcomes. (Rewards, revelations, damnations, etc.)

And yes folks, that 'more present attention' thing really *does* lead to an increase in appreciation for what you have.

Call it gratitude. Smelling those roses and all that. Because, rather than having a head and a heart full of obedience, approval seeking and apocalyptic terror, your senses have room for the details and pleasures of evening walks, eating lovely food and noticing the musical chatter of birds.

But no, it's not just the small things. Living for the sake of it absolutely lets you pursue grand, long term objectives – set yourself challenges, go to extremes, discipline yourself to endure and, if you choose, author your own life meaning stories. To say to yourself: even though I know it's all pointless, I elect to make *this* my point because I bloody well like the sound of it.

Once again, balance is key. Becoming your own chastising god or narrowing your options too vigorously will almost certainly *not* increase your potential for happiness – and in fact making the 'just because' belief portfolio pay off requires honesty and awareness as much as it does gratitude and fearlessness. However, once you begin to invest in this existential stock, you will soon discover that it comes with a set of very simple self-correcting levers, an inherent philosophical homeostasis mechanism. In fact, living just for the sake of it pretty well guarantees that you won't be locking yourself into ideological straitjackets or missions, and so the inevitable rolling tweaks and fine tunings required to keep your happiness potential high can happen with much less resistance and no punitive judgement or bullying threats.

And as for the inevitable setbacks, mostly you can just shrug them off or, if you're like me, make art out of them. At the very least you can prevent them from traumatising you permanently or stranding you in paranoia and mistrust, because now you know that in the end nothing matters. There is no plan, no great secret and no special role for you in destiny's dire and didactic drama. Life just happens. You're just here. Now. Reading this. From this point on you are free to do whatever you want.

LIVING LIGHTLY

We've all heard that saying about treading lightly on the earth. Figuratively speaking, we can also tread lightly on ourselves – and this is what the meaningless lifestyle makes it easier to achieve. Thus, whilst we may ignore all the noises of external control, it also behoves us well to use a soft touch on ourselves.

Naturally I am not advising you to slide into a bog of ill-disciplined slovenliness, not because I think it's intrinsically bad or wrong but because in my experience it doesn't appear to deliver enough happiness. (By all means, beg to differ if it works for you, though.) What I am suggesting however is that when it comes to those long term ambitions or big picture meanings – and indeed the very stories you tell yourself about who you are – a kind of quantum vagueness is best. Have *some* co-ordinates but not all. Err on the side of the general rather than the specific. Go plural. Have two or three or forty two points and as many personalities as you like. Why just be plain old mono Roberta when you can have much more fun as 5.1 surround sound Robbie, Bobby and Berta as well? Also, be prepared to sacrifice any or all sacred cows should better options arise or radical uncertainty intervene. The universe isn't fixed, so why would you want to be?

Imagine you have an existential compass. It will always show you due north, and therefore allow you to see where you are in relation, but this compass also lets you change where north is. Sure, there are still handy poles to help with orientation but now you are able to move them around. After all, you are ground zero in the universe of your life, so you get to decide where the axes are and when and where to finesse their positioning. Or throw them out altogether and start again. Or not, as you see fit.

It doesn't fucking matter. The *Pointless Revolution* liberates you from all that reductionist, linear, right/wrong, sacred mission bullshit. So, just as you may well reject all those socially ordained visions for you and your life – spiritual, consumerist, customary, etc – it's perfectly okay for you to jettison your own internalised must imperatives and higher purposes and just *be*.

One thing's for sure, you certainly don't need my permission.

PS:

Consider this: by suggesting that the universe exists because it wants to know itself, or indeed that its telos is self-knowing or self-becoming, are we not effectively saying something very much like: the universe exists just because, or *for the sake of it?* In fact what other reason could there be? After all, the universe (God, existence, etc) has nothing to prove and cannot refer to externalities for validation, guidance or assessment. Thus, even if we do concede that self-knowing is a reason/point/objective what we're really saying is that the reason for existence is that it gets on and exists. Indeed, that existence *is* a reason – or something equally tautologous. Perhaps, in the end, the most divine higher purpose is simply to be like the universe and just be.

9.
ETHICAL INVESTMENT
IN A MEANINGLESS VOID

or

Why not to be a total bastard
(even though it doesn't really matter)

Morality – or if you prefer, a basic decency – is a form of currency. Like money, which is a universally transferable credit mechanism or token of transactional trust, ethics are our cultural, philosophical and psychological credit facility.

In this chapter (which, in a way, is a lengthy disclaimer) I discuss our evolved sociability and capacity for empathy, and suggest that these factors can underwrite a risk/reward position that, sensibly applied, urges us towards ethical behaviours without recourse to Essentialist control and punishment mechanisms. In other words, goodness for the sake of it.

U ncomfortable truth time.

The trouble with all this freedom and empowerment stuff is that it can manifest itself in forms of arrogance. Likewise, the 'pointless p.o.v.' can encourage some to veer towards a self-centredness that too easily morphs into righteousness, a lack of care for others and sometimes into outright cruelty and abuse. Too often I have heard self-appointed spiritual truth warriors blithely dismiss suffering and injustice. They trot out apparently enlightened ideological excuses like:

- It's their karma – so therefore they deserve to be poor, crippled or trafficked into sex slavery, and it's perfectly fine for me to stand by and do nothing because it's *my* karma to be a wealthy, entitled light being.

- The universe (or God) is testing them – ah, so *that's* why they were sexually abused at the age of ten or stepped on a landmine.

- Oh, she's just one of the sheeple – she's not awakened like us – she won't make the cut when the apocalypse comes – forget her.

- It's your fault – hey, I got the dharma, buddy, so if you missed out it's because you're stupid, lazy or you got the wrong 'tude, dude.

    +

- So what, man, none of this shit matters anyway – which means I can rape that bitch, rip these stupid suckers off, shovel pollution into the atmosphere, party till the end of time – fucken whatever, etc.

Lurid examples aside, let's be frank; disavowing oneself of the dictats of the parental/external and shedding the baggage of Essentialist tropes does not necessitate nice. Indeed, the meaningless lifestyle is avowedly amoral. Not only does it come without rusted on codes of behaviour but it tends to regard all ethics as anthropogenic and environmental – as an evolved, pragmatic response to the ever-present problem of balancing individual desire and group cohesion. By contrast, liberating ourselves from slave narratives and reductionist meaning stories doesn't mean we will *inevitably* become arseholes. Indeed, we remain entirely free to choose kindness, compassion, humility and gratitude; not because we *have to* but because we *can*.

So, even if many (or indeed most) people continue to operate from a kind of poor me/poison world default setting, and are deeply entrenched in self-defeating behaviour patterns, does this give the rest of us licence to turn a blind eye or lapse into punishing 'we know better' selfishness and wanton brutality?

Perhaps you can already guess my position on this – but I'm not here to bore you with yawnsome 'be nice' platitudes or messianic mountaintop sermons. Rather, what I'd like to suggest is an ethical portfolio based on the risk/reward architecture of existential economics. And yes, much of what follows is (hopefully) obvious. In fact, to be honest, I'm only writing this chapter in case any of you take my 'do whatever you want' philosophy as a green light for uncaring nastiness and/or righteous entitlement – or indeed to crudely essentialise others on the basis of their ethnicity, gender, sexuality, postcode, choice of trousers or taste in music. Furthermore, I would like to unambiguously declare that *The Pointless Revolution* does not endorse any dystopian conspiracies, solipsistic spiritual arrogance, left/right paranoias, 'world gone mad' victim whinges, divine higher purposes, chosen people exceptionalism, system blaming cop outs or 'meant to be' capitulations. (Got that?)

Freedom, as I have argued, comes with responsibility and, I would add, with an entirely practical call to action regarding the welfare of others. None of us exists in a vacuum (physically or psychologically). We exist within a societal framework that not only informs our very sense of identity but makes possible and helps to sustain our endeavours. Therefore, just as we might choose to live for the sake of it, I believe it behoves us well to choose to be moral for the sake it – because the ethical investment strategy also pays out dividends in happiness; let alone raw survival.

SOCIAL SIMIANS R US

More potentially disconcerting truth.

Humanity has no particular or specially ordained right to exist. Sure, we think we're the exception and we can clearly differentiate ourselves from all other Earthly lifeforms – opposable thumbs, abstract thought, indie rock, sourdough bread – but we are just one of many species sharing this planet. Even though we are the current apex predator, we too rely on our ability to remain in sync with the biosphere, and upon having enough nous not to extinguish ourselves in either error or in an orgy of cannibalising violence. Just like mice or locusts, if we breed up too big we will burn up our food sources. Likewise, if the demands we place upon the environment outstrip supply, we will be left with two stark choices. Adapt or die. Or find another planet to exploit.

And of course, as I discussed way back in Chapter 1, we separate ourselves from what we call nature as part of the central denial – our individual and cultural refusal to accept our mortal animality. By doing this we blind ourselves to one of the most fundamental aspects of our humanity; namely, that we are a *social* species. When right wing ideologues like the late British Prime Minister Margaret Thatcher declare that there is no such thing as society, they are elevating the denialist reflex into the sanitised stratosphere of academic and political theorising. Indeed, the cult of the individual that we in the West have been incrementally enshrining since the advent of industrialisation can also be regarded as part of a broadly based desire to pretend we're not really social animals. That we don't live in co-dependent and mutually beneficial relationship with one another and, by extension, the rest of the biosphere.

Seen through the lens of evolution, sociability is one of a number of successful adaptations. Herd cohesion is a survival mechanism. The pooling and sharing of individual effort, knowledge and ability allows social animals (especially mammals) to divide 'labour' and share learning, thereby enabling them to deal more effectively with a wider range of environmental threats, better protect their young and ultimately to pass on their genes. (In addition, social technologies like language and symbolic representation have allowed our species to archive both individual and shared knowledge *outside* of our brains, in a kind of communally accessible external hard drive.)

As a corollary, homo sapiens, like other social animals, evolved a set of group behavioural rules to maximise the synergistic benefits of herd living. Then, as our species further refined tools like language and began to invent increasingly abstract modes of engaging with each other and the world – art, gods, agriculture, trade, centralised state power, etc – those very same group survival adaptations became abstracted into what we recognise as morality and custom. What began as something avowedly nature based and survivalist like 'co-operate effectively or get eaten by lions or murdered by other humans' segued gradually into the more modern sounding 'follow these divinely or kingly ordained dictats or go to hell, get executed, be imprisoned or find yourself banished.' The de-coupling of morality from core survival is, however, simply a sleight of hand. A kind of intellectual alchemy. A disinfected rebranding of evolutionary imperative. Now we're not merely surviving, we're being *good*. Or conversely, *bad*.

This is not to say that humans living in pre-agricultural clan societies didn't have individual desires or indeed compete with one another for power, prestige and the most fertile mates. Not for one minute am I lauding some kind of nomadic utopia – but I am suggesting that the basis of modern morality is entirely rooted in practicality. At their core, ethics are a response to a problem.

- What is the most agreeable and effective balance between the desires of the individual and the smooth functioning of the tribe – how can we gain the maximum benefit from both the drive and ability of the one and the synergies of the many?

And for the individual:

- To what extent, if any, does the pursuit of my own objectives trump the benefits I accrue from being part of society – how can I best negotiate the compromise between my rights and responsibilities?

Indeed, when considered as an evolutionary adaptation, morality is a cost/benefit framework, a negotiated settlement between desire and the consequences of its pursuit. A risk mitigation strategy for group living. An evolving set of behaviour management and impulse control levers intended to optimise outcomes for the players *and* the team.

Other than keeping us alive, physically safe, psycho-emotionally functional, and underwriting the ongoing viability of the herd, I would argue that ethics serve no other beneficial purpose. Their entanglement with the command and control narratives of the parental/external authority complex has resulted in the kind of simplistic good/bad distinctions that support power elites and ideologues – and, as observed throughout history, have been regularly employed to legitimise all manner of violent and prejudicial crusades, to entrench both privilege and disadvantage, and to prop up notions of normalcy and deviance. In group/out group dichotomies and the sometimes genocidal mania they make allowable would almost certainly be impossible without the arbitrary self-declared imprimatur of 'rightness'.

That said, those acting on moral impulses have also fought successfully for the widening of what is sometimes called 'the circle of empathy'. Things that were once unremarkable (or at least tolerated) are now either unthinkable or definitively frowned upon – public execution, wife beating, cruelty to animals and so on. Indeed, since I was a teenager in the 1980s, we here in Australia have gone from routine, virtually unquestioned cultural homophobia to embracing the right of gay and transgender people to marry (all this in spite of the Luddite protestations of bible bashers and the hysterical paranoia of right wing conspiracy theorists).

In my view, both these historical trends, to either oppress or liberate, underline the bedrock function of morality – to bolster group cohesion and moderate the destructive excesses of individual self-interest. Like any tool, ethics can be used to build up or destroy, conserve or reform. To argue for the maintenance of custom or to advocate for change. The ongoing tug-o-war is society's way of arriving at a workable compromise, of balancing out the frequently competing urges of sub-groups and individuals within the greater tribe. And we do this because society *works* for us, individually and collectively.

Whoa – hold up there. What do you mean society works?

Yes, I know I have spent a lot of time railing against societal forces and their negative, disempowering impact on our individual lives. However, I have also consistently acknowledged that I wouldn't be writing this if it wasn't for a supporting architecture of prevailing socio-economic and, dare I say it, political conditions. Whatever criticisms we may level at the herd and its institutions it would be disingenuous, if not downright fallacious, to deny that we seriously depend upon the accrued knowledge and ongoing coherence of the society we find ourselves in. Cue the clichés: standing on the shoulders of giants, resting in the arms of my community, etc.

No matter how unique and non-conformist you think you are – trailblazer, soul rebel, iconoclast – it is abundantly clear that you owe a large part of your survival, sanity and skill sets to the complex web of relationship that binds couples, families and communities together. Indeed, as I argued in the previous chapter, language itself is a social technology.

Finally, it is worth briefly reiterating that our very identity itself is, to a large extent, socially constructed:

- Initially imbibed and refined via the infant/toddler interactions we have with our parents and others.
- Further rehearsed and moulded as school aged children through our emerging relationships with friends, classmates, teachers and sports coaches.
- Influenced further still by referral to cultural norms reflected in media, the arts and other socially-authored narratives.

True, we also learn to bite back – developing distinctly idiosyncratic traits, learning to refuse and pursuing personal interests – but even as the evolving I/Not I feedback loop matures into a detailed and consistently recognisable adult identity, we still find ourselves deeply and profoundly enmeshed in a foundational relationship with others. What better reason do we need to care about one another?

THE ECONOMICS OF GIVING A SHIT

As people wedded to a broader community and, presumably, with a network of friends, loved ones and colleagues, it is apparent to most of us that our best self-interest is served by both wishing others well and treating them with respect. The oft-used term 'enlightened self-interest' covers this adequately. In other words, I will prosper by doing what I can to help others prosper and, more generally, if the wider society in which I live is viable, functional and plural enough to allow me the scope to indulge my various proclivities and walk around without an oppressive fear of murder, rape and abduction.

In the political-economic sphere we can refer to this as the social contract. Although this term originated with Enlightenment philosopher Jean-Jacques Rousseau (and, in particular, his 1762 work *Du contrat social ou Principes du droit politique*), we can understand it broadly as a framework of laws and institutions that formalise and adjudicate the relationship between the state and the citizenry. Or, to put it another way, a deal that says 'in return for obeying laws, paying taxes and surrendering the right to use violence as and when I may, the sovereign will provide me with

Choice & morality

As I argued way back in Chapter 2, morality, in its 'purest' form, can only really exist in the context of free choice. We can only be moral if we are also able to be immoral. Obvious though this sounds, in my experience it is one of those 'hidden in plain sight' things that most people I know routinely overlook. Instead, they defer to the 'had to' belief. It was their duty and so on. For instance, someone recently said to me, 'Oh well, all this 'be free' stuff is okay for single guys like you but for blokes like me it's a bit more complicated. I have kids.' Pulling this apart, what we get to is the commonplace narrative of obligation; as though the fact of his kids means the dad in question has no choice. To be brutal, this is false. He *does* have a choice. He can leave the family, give the kids up for adoption or otherwise neglect and victimise them. (After all, it's not like this sort of stuff doesn't happen. Family violence and child abuse is hardly unheard of, so clearly a bunch of folks *are* choosing differently from our dutiful dad.) Far from being trivial, banal or dismissive, I believe this is fundamental and can create a powerful understanding.

Why do I say this? Because, as many children later come to attest, ubiquitous parental obligation mantras so often morph into resentment, control (to page 127)

physical security, agreeable socio-cultural conditions, impartial rule-based dispute resolution mechanisms and useful shared assets like roads and stuff.' Whatever we may think of the particulars – specific laws, certain people in power, the role of central banks – the fact remains that there exists, explicitly and implicitly, an agreement that slices up and apportions the various individual and collective rights and responsibilities. However flawed you think the current model is, (indeed, even if you believe it's fundamentally fucked), its base level function is to engender and maintain conditions for private desire and public benefit to co-exist.

Drilling down into the more concrete realm of inter-personal relations, a similar 'contract' operates. The banal fact is that we mostly agree to get along and to respect one another's boundaries because being a totally selfish cunt will typically leave us on the outer – friendless, reviled and liable to be left to stew in our own juices. Reap what you sow and all that.

Okay, I know this is grindingly obvious and I apologise for appearing to descend into territory normally reserved for mawkish sentimental memes and vomitous Hollywood, tissue box crud. I most certainly am *not* here to preach family values or huggy bear hippiedom. After all, life is ultimately meaningless and nothing *really, truly* matters – and the vast majority of socially sanctioned narratives and imperatives are simplistic, reductionist modes of control built upon a bedrock of fear and denial.

So, why bother being moral? Why give any ground whatsoever to others? In fact, if it wasn't for the risk of getting caught, why

(from page 126) and guilt tripping. *If only you knew what I had to go without* and other such complaints. How many mums lost their figures and gave up their careers? How many dads worked ten days a week so you could have a roof over your head? How many couples tell their kids, *after all we've done for you, you should blah blah blah*? (My guess is that many of you will be familiar with this.) In my view, these punishing narratives are a side effect of feeling obliged. Trapped. Thus, in a way, the famed parental sacrifice story and others of its ilk are not truly moral. Rather, they are tales of obedient repetition, of meeting herd-approved and highly ritualised expectations. Or, in the case of religion, an example of cravenly caving in to a petulant God who wants you to honour their astonishing godliness by 'worshipping' them and doing whatever they tell you – unless of course you prefer eternal hellfire or coming back as a bug.

In saying this I am in no way scorning parenthood or downplaying the enormity and relentlessness of child rearing – nor indeed seeking to castigate you for choosing to make personal sacrifices for loved ones – but I *am* suggesting that by de-coupling ourselves from notions of obligation, and accepting that we *do* have free choice, we can begin to counter and minimise the frequently debilitating and 'unhappy making' sense of treadmill, duty and self-denial so common in human societies. I feel sure that far fewer of us would kick the dog if we felt that we weren't also being systemically kicked.

Boorishly technical and/or semantic though this may seem, I would argue that it is much less about the pedantic honing of definitions than it is about a psycho-emotional re-aligning of motivation. What is it that drives my choice to sacrifice for those I love? Am I just being a good boy and hoping for gold stars? Do I want my kindnesses to be repaid? Glorified? Deified? Or rather, do I 'behave' because the price of misbehaviour is too high? To me, none of these seems especially ethical. Pragmatic, savvy and the lesser of two evils but *not* moral. Nor a result of truly empowered choice. Ultimately, what this all points to is our near universal tendency to defer to externally mandated measures. Again, if this capitulation really made us happy, I'd go with it – but in my observation the most common lived experience of the 'had to' narrative is that of feeling shackled and, in turn, resentful, stymied, silenced and unappreciated (and, by extension, the acting out behaviours that go with it). And so the cycle goes on and on and on.

would any of us be law abiding members of our given communities? Why, for instance, don't we abandon the formalism and niceties of civil society and agree to live in an ungoverned free-for-all where each of us is perfectly free to steal, kill, rape and enslave?

In my experience there are three key and regularly payable dividends that flow from an 'ethical investment' strategy:

- Genuinely care for and behave respectfully around others and, largely, they will return the favour – it's a quid pro quo kinda thing – love and be loved, etc.
- Operating ethically greatly contributes to feelings of self-worth and overall happiness – look yourself in the mirror, sleep at night, live without crushing guilt/shame, etc.

     +

- Vastly improved odds of continued survival and physical security – the confidence to go about your business without the hyper-vigilance and weaponry required to defend life, limb and loved ones from random assault – ability to live in pleasant, easy-going surroundings, as opposed to heavily fortified bunkers.

The first and third are hopefully obvious to you and (thank fuck) we shall now put them to bed. It's the second one that's the real kicker. That sense we all have of ourselves as either a 'good' or 'not so good' person is pivotal to the way we think of ourselves – the story we all tell ourselves about our overall character and the manner in which we act out in pursuit of our objectives. Almost without exception we like to believe that we're a good person and that we operate in a fashion informed by a suite of well-considered values. Furthermore, we tell ourselves that these values are rooted in some kind of 'logic' or basic sense and that, taken as a whole, they fall into the 'good' category (even if we sometimes knowingly do bad things). In fact it's difficult to imagine how anyone could sustainably operate in the genuine belief that they were bad, rotten to the core or evil. As we have noted, even those wont to participate in wholesale slaughter find ways to convince themselves they are acting in the service of the good.

It is of course this very desire – to feel like a good person, to be able to live with oneself – that makes all those externally ordained good/bad mantras so powerful. Because morality is so intrinsically subjective we can only ever *hope* we're being good, which is why we look so feverishly for confirmation/validation in external sources of moral authority like religion, custom and ideology. *If I do as Siddhārtha says that will surely make me good. Won't it?* Thus, the parent pleasing reflex and our evolved need for herd acceptance makes us easy prey for the spinners of moral sophistry.

Whilst conspiracy paranoiacs will insist that this is proof of a fiendish, worldwide plot involving commercial newsmedia, chem trails and shadowy Jewish banking families, their so-called analysis is informed not only by a staggering historical amnesia but by an addiction to the slave narrative fantasies of righteous victimhood and impending apocalypse. In addition, like so many in our denialist culture, they ignore animal fact. Clearly, as social creatures, we are hardwired to want to fit in and, in addition, we primates are well known for our imitative tendencies, for our 'learning by mimicry' skills. Thus, following the leader and taking our cues from others (herd mentality) pre-date the agricultural revolution, let alone the Vatican, the Rothschilds or gay marriage legislation.

So, dystopian conflations and meaningless voids aside, we have a vested interest in appearing to ourselves and others as good. Indeed, I would contend that this goes right to the heart of who we think we are and the kind of life we wish to live.

To use myself as an example, even though I've spent decades carefully extricating what I now regard as 'my true self' from the slurry of parental/external musts, shoulds and oughta be's, I too cling to the idea that I am basically good. Moral, principled, etc. What's more, this remains the case in spite of my preference for not believing too much or too strongly. (Yes, even nihilists care.)

However, I would be lying if were to suggest that I arrived at this via a careful, economic risk metrics process. Indeed, like most everybody, I was a sucker for all manner of ideological, self-righteous, egomaniacal prattle. I just *assumed* my ethics were sound – *of course they were*. I *asserted* the superiority of my various stances based on a bunch of habitual assumptions. However, age saw me shed the baggage of belief bit by bit until I landed, in my late forties, at the threshold of liberation, of the deepest, most broadly based happiness I have ever known. And a critical part of that equation is the feeling I still get that, on the whole, I'm an alright kinda guy.

Yet, when I peel the layers back further, what I find is a self-serving wish for the world to operate in a civil, law abiding, non-violent manner; because I know that in a lawless state I would quickly be either captured or killed by much stronger men with guns or, at the very least, no longer be afforded the freedom and cultural conditions to live a life of peaceful, indulgent, largely barefoot bohemia. I most certainly would *not* be sitting here, with no immediately apparent means of defence, pouring my time into writing relatively arcane nonsense like this with unlocked doors and music playing loudly enough to mask the sound of approaching goons. In short, it's about trust.

A quick cost/benefit analysis reveals a much better flow of happiness dividends from relationships based on trust. Societal, clan or family relationships founded on mistrust, fear and paranoia strike me as a truly awful investment. Imagine the colossal expenditure in nervous energy, firearms and electric perimeter fencing required to maintain life and liberty in a truly dog eat dog world. I mean, fuck, it's just not worth it. We're all gonna die anyway so, in the interim, we may as well all have the most rewarding and fascinating time we possibly can; as opposed to lives scarred by constant wariness and a hugely increased likelihood of rape, torture and peonage followed by a violent, agonising death.

Morality – or if you prefer, a basic decency – is a form of currency. Like money, which is a universally transferable credit mechanism or token of transactional trust, ethics are our cultural, philosophical and psychological credit facility. They underpin our individual and collective confidence to plan for the future; to take the risks involved in co-operative ventures, to drive our cars in the reasonable expectation of safe arrival, and to buy cream buns from the local patisserie without first having to check for sneakily concealed razor blades. Not to mention the formation of loving and intimate bonds – or relationships likely to support the creation and successful rearing of children.

Seriously, can it *be* any more obvious?

THE BENEFITS OF SELECTED COMPLIANCE

For those of you cringing at my use of the term 'basic decency' – which I confess is as oxymoronic as that other ludicrously stupid catch-all: common sense – I have employed it deliberately to point at one of the core psycho-social strategic behavioural quandaries confronting every member of the tribe:

- When, to what extent, and under which conditions, is it best to conform?

More particularly, how can we square our Existentialist notions of pointlessness and our general rejection of commonplace slavethink with the realpolitik of gaining the advantages of social acceptance and maintaining valuable friendships?

Any attempt to answer this question with hardline rules or sweeping pre-judgement is at the very least lazy, quite likely stupid, and perhaps even a fear driven and futile mode of control. As I have argued throughout, retreating into a sandpit of neat, encapsulated rules is an infantile response to a complex, ever changing world. All of which leaves us on our own when it comes to deciding how much of our hard won freedom is predicated on topically applied tinctures of compliance.

Stripping out sanctimony and sentiment, even the more misanthropic amongst us can surely employ smart tactics. Smart because it is plain to see that for the reward of ongoing, sustainable happiness there is a cost – and the price is sometimes politeness, etiquette, deference, etc. Sometimes even judicious silence and the temporary tolerating of utter fuckwits. (For instance, I occasionally endure meetings with marketing types, nodding and trying to smile at their vile, dehumanising garbage. Sure, I often need to sneak off and throw up after hearing them say 'touch point' and 'audience engagement' ad nauseum, but y'know, I'm thinkin' long term. Or trying to anyway.)

So, even though I've been extolling the virtues of meaningless living and doing whatever you want, there is this thing called balance; or perspective. To be fair, not *all* social norms are spirit crushing impositions. Most sane people don't actually *want* to anally penetrate small children or defecate in restaurants. Yes, waiting politely in line can sometimes be irritating and listening to grandpa's brain-freezingly dull yarns for the 4000th time can test your patience to breaking point, but we grin and bear it because, well, there's a bigger picture. This too shall pass, choose your battles, don't sweat the small shit, and so on.

In terms of advantage accrued, it is moot whether we actually *feel* moral or just *act* it. Some might say 'gee, that's heartless' but I would counter by pointing out that every single person I have ever met, myself included, plays a role (or roles) in public. We may not like to admit it but we are all actors. Each of us is an ensemble cast, and we walk and talk a range of characters hopefully well suited to the scene we find ourselves in.

To conclude, selective conformity is not only a sign of genuinely free choice but, (coughs, shuffles uncomfortably), is plain old …

THE EMPATHY ELEPHANT

Amongst all this talk of cost/benefit we have so far left our capacity for empathy to one side. Regardless of whether we are emotionally compelled to be a nice person or we just coolly elect to act in an ethical manner, we have an evolved mechanism for knowing how others feel. Recent conjecture in neuroscience and neuro-psychology about mirror (or cubelli) neurons and our emerging understanding of brain function, although still hotly contentious, has pointed to a folio of biologically underwritten behavioural and psycho-emotional traits that pre-dispose us towards imitative abilities that include being able to mimic feeling states.

But of course it didn't take brain scanners to show us this. As a story-telling species we have long known the power of imagery, poetry, song and dance to transport us – to be so compelling that we cry, laugh and scream. Part of what makes film so powerful is we can place ourselves in the shoes of the people we see on the screen. That we feel what they feel.

Most of you, I'm sure, will recall those moments when you first began to *really* understand another's suffering. When you were first truly sorry that your actions hurt someone. In addition, you most likely remember times when you appealed to someone else's empathy – *can you imagine how that made me feel?*

While there are those who overplay or cynically exploit this card, and still others who indulge in the righteous self-seeking spectacle of guilt, the point I'm making is that empathy plays into morality. We feel compelled to limit the harm we do to others because it hurts us when we see the results of our actions. We can too easily imagine how we would react if the boot was on the other foot.

Here again we see the realities of sociability at play. If being cruel and excessively selfish leaves us feeling awful we are far less likely to be career arseholes. Moreover, it is often observed that psychopaths, sociopaths and people with what is called 'low EI' (emotional intelligence) lack empathy. They do not understand, or are able to plausibly deny, the impacts of their actions upon others.

In addition, things like the Holocaust are only possible when the victims are dehumanised. This is also why mechanised 'distance killing' like drone warfare is easier on the trigger pullers than having to stab or strangle their enemies one by one. Likewise, farmers of livestock warn against making pets of or naming favourite animals – and, to be blunt, how many of us in the cosy, over-weight West would eat meat as often, if at all, were we required to personally slaughter the pig for our pancetta?

Deliberate, calculated, ongoing viciousness and death dealing is, for the vast majority of us, only possible where there is a disconnect and/or abstraction. When empathy is not triggered.

The salient point here is that, no matter how ultimately nihilistic our view of life and the universe may be, or how thoroughly we abjure passively received middle class orthodoxies, our brain wiring will most likely prevent or countervail any lasting impulse we have to go on a killing spree, become a serial rapist or steal our best friend's iThings.

Therefore, although there are doubtless exceptions, it seems fair to suggest that abandoning the safety net of Essentialist meaning will *not* turn you into a total bastard – and furthermore, that those who insist it will are clinging to the levers of command and control and utilising the manipulative power of fear to blackmail you into persisting with their dumbed down, nursery rhyme, aspirin-addled fantasy of a nice, safe, neatly-ordered, anthropomorphised universe that kisses you nighty-night when you're good but sends you to your room forever if you step out of line.

Their way is be good or else.

The way I'm recommending is more like: if you choose to be good you'll probably really like it and, what's more, in the long run, it'll most likely pay off. So y'know, why wouldn't you?

CONFESSIONS OF A MIDDLE AGED, ARSE COVERING, EFFETE INTELLECTUAL

As indicated earlier, I have dedicated time to writing this chapter for what I confess are reasons that transcend the strictly intellectual. Not only do I personally have no desire to live in or inadvertently create the conditions for the emergence of a trust-free society, I want to reassure myself that I am making every attempt to minimise the risk of my words being co-opted by demagogues eager to legitimise their divide and conquer agendas.

I'll admit it – I am one of those uncalloused effetes with a skill set that could readily be categorised as somewhat 'soft'. Whilst I can write you a nifty critique of the latest contemporary dance sensation and direct your band's latest video, I would fail abysmally at building adequate shelter, hunting and skinning wild animals, hand-to-hand combat with knife wielding ninjas, and stitching up open wounds. I also have serious and well-founded doubts about my ability to survive very long in the wild or indeed my willingness to operate a machine gun in a pre-emptive strike against a would be terror cell. Speaking bluntly, I am what many of you would likely call useless. In fact, if you were to call me a lazy, indulged, white bourgeois hypocrite I would probably, in one of my more honest moods, largely agree with you.

Fortunately my attitude to these things is pretty much, *yeah, so fucking what*. I attach no moral or other significance to my apparent lack of real manliness and I do not buy into the dishonest pantomime of white middle class guilt. I am not ashamed or embarrassed by, nor will I apologise for, the fact of my being born male, in England, working class, short-sighted, left-handed, svelte and heterosexual. Neither will I claim special status because of these things. However, I *do* place real value on trust-based personal and social relationships. And that value is existential, emotional and economic. It also derives from the ample opportunities I presently have to pursue happiness without the need to dodge the Gestapo or resort to the use of guns to protect myself from random right wing pitchfork mobs.

Let there be no doubt – I most certainly extract enormous benefit from trust and empathy in my personal and vocational life and from the rule of law in the communal sphere. I choose to be moral because it darn well suits me to. And, of course, it feeds beautifully into the various narratives I have about myself. The story that I call Paul.

You will note that surplus to requirements in all this weighing up of pros and cons are those age old war horses:

- Gods, spirits and other numina – or the promises and threats of their associated afterlives.
- Customs, traditions and 'national character' tropes – dinkum Aussie, typical Pommie bullshit.
- Gender and sexuality stereotypes – tough man, dumb man, patriarchal rapist, fucking faggot, etc.
- Political and class ideologies.
- Destiny, karma and other reputedly spiritual imperatives.
- Attainments, trophies, trinkets of status, bucket lists, etc.
- Socially mandated notions of honour, worthiness, greatness, etc.

So yes, this chapter has, amongst other things, been a long form disclaimer, an exercise in fancily expressed arse coverage; because I have no wish for the items on the above list to dominate my life or yours. *The Pointless Revolution* is designed to set you free, to give you (almost) *carte blanche* to revel in the meaningless beauty and wonder of being alive.

When I consider the other available options in the marketplace and weigh them up in terms of how I might best invest my existential slush fund for maximum potential happiness, I know where my life dollars will flow. And what's more I trust that enough of you will be okay with that – and, who knows, maybe some of you may even join me on this gloriously pointless journey.

10.
THE AUTHENTICITY CHANNEL

or

Developing a really good bullshit detector

Just as we need not be the slaves of external signals, so too we are
not bound to be the victims of our own internal haranguing.
Our fears, our persecution complexes, the reflexive hankering
for herd approval – all of these can be challenged
and their power to drive habitual behaviour revoked.

In this chapter I address the problem of identifying the 'authentic' or 'true' inner voice/self. It is then with some irony that I resort to the listicle, outlining the broad brushstrokes in a '15 Things' format to help you get started on the process of sifting out the real you from the abundance of internalised external noise.

Throughout this book I have discussed at some length the 'co-entailed' phenomenon of the I and the Not I, the internal and the external. I have addressed the effects of externally ordained narratives and touched upon the social construction of identity. You will, I trust, have understood my basic position(s) on the personal and cultural impacts of what I call the parental/external authority complex. However, buried in the sub-strata is a fundamental and far less abstract challenge. As a close friend asked me recently: how can we disentangle our true inner voice from all the other noise?

It's a great question and it cuts to the practical heart of my endeavour here. Teasing it out a little further we get:

- How do I know I am making a genuinely free choice, as opposed to re-enacting the rituals of socially received dogma – or that I am making life choices based upon truly self-authored imperatives rather than defaulting to culturally sanctioned ideas about meaning, morality and attainment?
- How do I know I am no longer acting out the narratives and operating on the beliefs that others (parents and loved ones especially) have effectively imposed upon me – or that I have created a 'character' and arrived at a belief portfolio that is truly mine?

Or, deeper still:

- How can I tell when the identity I call me is finally mine – and not simply an internalised amalgam of external signals – a jumbled mirror of the other?
- How, in fact, can I recognise myself?

Naturally, these kinds of questions can take us down highly metaphysical rabbit-holes towards conundrums around the very nature of self and consciousness and, further still, into the classic realist/idealist debate and its sibling schism, duality or non-duality (multiplicity or oneness). Whilst these are endlessly fascinating to explore – and are indeed the source of much ideological posturing from philosophers, scientists and the various spiritual schools – they sit outside the scope of this book.

This is not to casually dismiss them, nor lazily avoid the complexities they infer; rather, my intention here is to focus on both the self and the world of our *experience*. For even though our best currently available models tell us that the consistent, solid and detailed picture of the world that our brains conjure for us does not necessarily accord with the *actual* universe, whatever the level and form of our so-called illusion, our experience *is* our experience. Whether partly imagined, utterly deluded or incomplete, we *do* experience stuff; and the continuum of our experience is what we typically regard as our life and our identity. Thus, even putative illusion contributes to our total experience and adds to our overall picture of self and world. In short, our experience is a sequence of awareness events. Incidents of information transfer. So, although we may have no way of perceiving the universe as it truly is, the fact is that the universe also includes our anthropogenic delusions. Includes the experience we call living and identity. Includes the sensation I am currently having of typing out words I thought of just then and the awareness/consciousness event of you reading them.

Free will & determinism

One of the truly great schisms in Western philosophy is the ongoing debate about free will and determinism. Do we truly have freedom of choice – genuine agency – or are we simply executing a pre-set mathematical and/or divine process? Is free will a delusion; a masterful evolutionary adaptation that creates a plausible and compelling fantasy of selfhood? Indeed, is the very spectacle of the conscious and self-identifying I simply a co-entailed, symbiotic outcrop of an underlying information exchange? Is the thing we know as our 'life' merely a stream of meta-data – a data process that data processes itself as it goes along? Error correcting for fitness. Incrementally adjusting in order to preserve the homeostasis of a complex informational feedback mechanism.

Clearly, none of us are in a position to answer with absolute certainty – although many of us continue to posit dogmatic responses. The take out here, for me at least, is that in lieu of a definitive ruling from the universe or an irrefutable argument from someone far cleverer than I, we are left to deal with the primacy of our lived experience. We *experience* self and, in turn, that self has the experience of regular choice making. True, a bunch of our apparently conscious decisions are driven by subconscious networks in our brains and the proclivities inscribed by DNA, but I think it's fair to say that we all *feel* like we have free will and *act* as though we do; even if loads of us freely choose to wed ourselves to herd-approved slavethink mantras and sinner/victim narratives. (to page 137)

Putting aside any spiritual or quantum mechanical quibbles we may have, let's at least allow that we are presently *experiencing* (or are aware of) a highly patterned data stream that manifests as an iterated identity complex (or self, or life) which is located within a world with which we interact and have relationship – and furthermore that this relationship (or data exchange) is foundational. In other words, that the I and Not I of our experience co-create themselves via an ongoing intricately patterned dialogue. I apologise to the hardcore idealists amongst you for breaching the purity of your oneness mantra but y'know, I am aiming at a modicum of functional pragmatism here, as opposed to being ideologically pristine or cosmically awakened. (Phew.)

And so, assuming that we are all human beings living out our limited time here on planet Earth, let's get back to our dot points – because it is fair to say that if we're ever going to successfully reject slave narratives and become fully fledged existential adults who are neither shit scared nor in denial about mortality, we need to develop mechanisms to kick start and evaluate our transition from apron strings to liberation. Whilst some of this is intellectual, the real spark for sustainable change and the increased potential for broadly based happiness burns deeper in the psyche. For it is one thing to accept a well-constructed argument, it's another to unearth the energy to do anything about it.

Indeed, I would be selling you short if I were to suggest that all you need do is read this book, sign off on a few nifty Existentialist ideas and robotically follow in my footsteps. It would also be false for me to suggest that the process is free of entrenched ambiguities and uncertainties. Maybe even flat out contradictions. This is life, after all, not a fairy tale.

That said, I believe there are a handful of disciplines and attitudes – some techniques – that can help us go forward with more clarity and far less punitive, debilitating judgement. Although they won't necessarily make it clear when and if you've 'succeeded' they will (like the PHI from Chapter 2) help you begin and, what's more, provide you with useful tracking mechanisms. Their 'telos' is to formalise and make less nebulous the act of beginning and, along the way, trigger the kind of compassionate but truthful self-assessment that can deepen and enrich the journey. (Sorry if that sounds a bit New Agey, but I'm sure you get the point.)

(from page 136) You might think this a sidestep but my response to that would be: even our delusions are real. In other words, my free will fantasy *exists*. My subjective viewpoint, my self-serving biases, the very illusion of the self I call Paul; all are happening here and now in the overall existence complex. So, just as historically wealthy and healthy Westerners contrive to convince themselves that they are being ritually oppressed by toxic masculinity or gender-non-binary thought police, so too we may continue in the delusion of free agency. Freedom, after all, is experienced as a feeling state. It is a *sense* we have that we are able to make topical and specific choices in pursuit of our objectives without onerous constraint. Indeed, the experiential phenomenon of free will may well be analogous to the very notion of the quantised human self. Or, to simplify further, both the self and the will are kinds of experience. The veracity or otherwise of that experience (awareness) may ultimately be irrelevant.

And now for an esoteric aside …

While the techniques hinted at above are of a more pragmatic nature, there is another potential and, dare I say, profound change agent waiting for us in the wings, in the realm we most often refer to as the spiritual. If you wish, you can even call it mystical or transcendent. This experience, or source of motivation, has nothing to do with the clatter and bang of the everyday world and defies all attempts to squeeze it into narrow, narrative channels. It renders all detail irrelevant and, of course, is almost impossible to distil into language. Basically, it is the deepest of deep backgrounds, the very canvas upon which the splatter of our existence is cast. It can be accessed (beheld, glimpsed, asymptotically approached) through contemplation and meditation, and also in moments of deep emotion. Things like music, dance, love, despair, beauty, the stars at night, the light, the silence, certain drugs and even the death of loved ones can open a window to it – pretty well whatever seems to take you 'out of yourself' and give you that wider or higher perspective. Although religions and other Essentialist spiritual traditions have tried to overwrite it with their deities, alpha meanings and didactic imperatives – by extension judging and controlling you – it does not have to be this way. Indeed, by refusing to reduce this experience to simplistic, linear anthropocentric 'understanding', we can return to Earth, so to speak, with a greatly enhanced sense of liberty, fearlessness and equanimity. For me at least this is what lies at the very core of my new found happiness. I have referred to it variously as the ecstasy of nothingness and the liberation of meaningless being. The Pointless Revolution *itself.*

Of course, mystical transcendent euphoria is not a pre-requisite. No spiritual practise is required to start doing whatever you want. However, it has been a factor for me* and may well be for you; so it would be remiss of me not to mention it

(* More of this in Appendix 3.)

THE CHANNEL SURFING CHALLENGE

As befits a book with 'doing whatever you want' as part of its subtitle, there is no way I'm going to start lecturing you about what and what not to do. After all, I only know what works for me and I cannot assume that the tweaks *I* used will work for you. Thus, there is no need to enrol in a self-improvement course, take up yoga, stop smoking dope or set fire to your television set – although of course you are perfectly free to do so if you desire.

In truth, the taking up or giving up of 'activities' is kinda beside the point. Our challenge, as my friend suggested, is to learn to recognise; to sift out the voice and objectives of our genuine, base level self from the learned, habituated stuff we've imbibed from our dealings with the world. Simply turning vegan, quitting your job or coming out of the closet won't necessarily achieve this.

Firstly, let us acknowledge that the idea of the unitary mind is a myth. Everyone I have ever spoken with about this readily admits to having a head full of voices. These channels sometimes work in sync, sometimes at odds with one another. Some are kinder, others rip us to shreds. Many repeat the mantras of our parents and the judgements of others. There are whip crackers who are never satisfied and always mark us down and more compassionate, encouraging voices. In addition, there are truth tellers and those who peddle the kind of plausible deniability that allows self-seeking bias and personal mythologies to flourish, even to our detriment. Some of you, like me, will have voices that seem to be little boys or teenage girls, lyrical poets or BBC sports commentators. They might even have names. Let's face it, folks, it's a fucking racket in there; so much so that it has tempted many to deride 'the mind' altogether (a righteous ideological pose which is, of course, a by-product of the very mind these folks are supposedly rising above).

And yet, amidst the cacophony of judgement, addiction and denial, there is a quieter, steadier channel. This is 'the you that is always you', that sense you have that behind the spectacle of ego and the numerous dramas of emotion, ambition and conflict there is a continuous, bedrock I or me. It is the self that watches self. The point that views. The paradoxical core of our being: the maker and the made. (Insert further pretty phrasing here to suit.)

Some will call this the higher self, others the voice of the heart or instinct and still others the spirit, soul or God voice. Ultimately the label doesn't matter. Whatever the language, *this* is the voice, the you I am referring to.

NB:

Should you have absolutely no idea what I'm talking about here, the following will be of no or very limited use to you. Sorry.

For the rest of us, having identified that such a voice exists, the trick is to tune in and amplify it. To have it available at will to cut through the thickets of noise. To translate its vague, almost mystical whisperings into useful, practical clarity that can be carried through into the more mundane, everyday realm. To bring it down from the mountaintop retreat to the supermarket checkout queue. After all, what use is a supposedly higher consciousness if for the most part you continue to live a daily life ruled by slavethink, poison world paranoia and an incessant need to achieve, achieve, achieve?

Right then – let's fish out the remote, rig up the antenna and tune in.

Whilst things like 'me time', beautiful scenery and downshifting may well be conducive, they are just three of any number of external tweaks that can help clear away the frazzle and clutter. Even distancing yourself from tyrants, abusers and drama queens is just another instance of existential renovation, of altering the external furniture. In the long run these surgeries often devolve to mere moments or phases. Much like a smoker might try several times, using a different approach on each occasion, before successfully quitting. Ultimately, cosmetic tinkering alone is unlikely to get you into clear contact with your truest inner compass and deliver those lasting happiness returns. (Not strictly impossible perhaps but certainly a very long shot.)

For the vast majority it is a combination of external *and* internal reform and experimentation – taken together – that will more likely tune us into this voice. Furthermore, I would argue that to commit the common error of championing the internal (working on yourself) over the altering of your external circumstances is simply to impose yet another layer of orthodoxy. Remember, we're not on a virtuous enlightenment path here. This is much less about vibrating ourselves to heavenly superbness and far more about being happier and freer *now*. On Earth. So yeah, do the deep reflecting stuff by all means but don't forget to readjust that work/life balance and ditch the fuckwit boyfriend while you're at it. Because identifying the true voice (self, spirit, etc) takes practise – like twiddling the dial on your granny's analogue radio.

Thus, for what it's worth, here are the fifteen core techniques – intellectual, attitudinal, psycho-emotional, practical – that put me in direct, powerful and liberating contact with my innermost voice. I realise they represent only *my* experience and, what's more, that I am not a therapist, life coach or any kind of guru. (Please note: this list is not complete and what follows are the broad brushstrokes as best I can generalise them in a handy listicle format.)

1: Interview yourself – the Q&A method – a therapy sesh in your head.

Set up a formal dialogue, either in your head or out loud, in which one voice asks the questions and the other answers. For me, this typically takes the form of an imaginary press interview, with a little bit of therapy thrown in – like a cross between *HardTalk* and *In Treatment*. Basically, find a Q&A format that is familiar and makes sense for you. The trick is to keep asking why, how, etc and to answer with fearless honesty. Indeed, anything less than complete frankness is, in my view, a waste of time.

I have found that going on walks or taking nice long baths can create the time and space for this process to occur. In addition, I have found it useful to be quite structured and to focus on particular behaviours or emotional responses. Without being too rigid about it, it has proved beneficial for me to have an objective; usually to drill down into and gain a clearer understanding of my dysfunctional/habitual behaviours and emotional dramas and, thereafter, to create an awareness that makes happiness inducing change more possible.

Ultimately, the core objective is increased and honest self-awareness, and the linking of that heightened awareness to both external and internal behaviour change.

Useful questions include: What is the pattern here? What is the underlying objective of this behaviour? Why did you react like that? Where did you learn *that* narrative? What is your rationale for behaving like that? What is the feeling state you think this behaviour will engender?

2: Be absolutely honest – no sacred cows – no denial.

Underpinning the Q&A process is a ruthless commitment to honesty. This is the self laid bare – but remember, no one else need ever know. If you can feel yourself blocking, being evasive or making excuses, double down. (Why are you trying to avoid this?) However, if it really *is* too much right now, tag it for further examination and come back to it when you feel safer or more able to deal with the fallout.

In addition, your honesty radar should also be on the lookout for unnecessary drama and, of course, paralysis by analysis. Both are forms of evasion.

What I'm hinting at here is that honesty itself can be learned. Honed. Refined. It has many impersonators but the steady process of identifying and neutralising these imposters is what ultimately reveals the true voice.

3: Learn to recognise your own patterns and addictions – observe yourself without fear or favour.

With an honesty process in motion, it's time to pay particular attention to pattern recognition. Fortunately, the human brain is a genius at patterns. After all, it's how we render the world navigable and form consistent notions of self and character. Once we better understand our own patterned responses we create a valve of choice – because patterns can change and addictions can be overcome.

4: Develop a method for catching yourself in the loop and bringing decision making into the light.

Having started to notice our patterns, the next trick is to create a formal mechanism for hitting the pause button and asking ourselves whether we want to continue down well worn paths or try out different approaches. What this does is to formalise and make directly conscious the act of choice. The moment of decision then becomes less opaque, something we can take direct and undeniable responsibility for and, as a result, we become much less of a 'mystery' to ourselves.

Personally, I have found questions like this useful: Okay Paulie, now that we're here again, which way do we wanna go? Do we really believe that the same old/same old will deliver a better result? Or indeed, does this pattern actually serve us well?

Whichever way I respond and choose to move forward, I am left in no doubt that I am 100% responsible and, furthermore, that I made my choice freely.

5: Avoid self-punishment – catch those judgemental urges early.

Punishment and pejorative, getting down on yourself, generally don't inspire sustainable change or underwrite lasting happiness. Relentlessly chiding and whipping will simply serve to build up a store of resentment and resistance and create a pattern of continued failure and disappointment. And remember, all those so-called values and 'good person, good life' objectives are arbitrary. Humans *invented* them. Codified them. Shoved them down your throat.

We all have behaviours or 'flaws' that we are not proud of or wish we could alter but imposing socially approved punishment narratives on ourselves will only exacerbate the naughty child dynamic and/or fuel self destructive psycho-drama.

So, challenge those judgemental voices. Nip their controlling mantras in the bud.

6: Remind yourself often that none of this makes you a better person – be humble.

Just as punishment is a bad strategy, so too is delusional self-aggrandisement. Increasing your happiness potential and identifying your authentic inner voice is not about being 'better'. Forget hell, forget heaven, pay no heed to the cuddly god fantasy that high fives you when you die and says, 'dude, awesome personing down there.' The objective isn't external approval, it's increasing the odds of living the life you want.

So remember humility – and be alert to the traps and conceits of righteousness.

7: Remind yourself that none of this matters in the end – cos you're gonna die.

After all, sooner or later everything you did and said and all your glittering monuments to yourself will be as nothing. As good, bad, happy or sad as you are, or try to become, you and everyone you know will be just as dead as everyone else. This thought alone can often be enough to dissolve all the nagging tensions around right/wrong, doing well/not so well, etc. All striving is ultimately meaningless and all our control mechanisms fundamentally futile. So just fucking let it go.

Counter-intuitive though it may seem, you can actually *practise* letting go, just as you can alter other patterns of behaviour. Utilise the mechanisms outlined in point 4 to bring the choice making moment into the light. Remember, things like 'holding on' and control dramas are only habits – desires and behaviours we have learned – not immutable laws. Indeed, your psycho-emotional routines are as impermanent and inessential as everything else and, in the light of universally meaningless flux, may as well work *for* you as against you.

8: Catch yourself in approval seeking behaviour and prompt yourself to desist.

To illustrate this, I'll use myself as an example. In front of the mirror one morning I caught myself in compulsive preening behaviours. Why are you doing this, Paulie? I wondered. The honest answer was for the approval of the gorgeous young women who staff my fave local café. Then it occurred to me just how *much* time and effort I had invested into the seeking of female approval (and all for a fairly abysmal return, it must be said). From there it was easy to see how I was mired in mostly unconscious approval seeking behaviour – not just with the ladies but in work situations, with my buddies and, in fact, all over the bloody shop. I wanted everyone to think I was *soooo* fucking impressive; cool, smart, funny, you name it.

Since that pivotal morning in the bathroom I have set up a flagging habit – if this is about the approbation of others, stop. Now! *Right now!*

And I'm here to tell you it works. The time I plough into external approval has reduced in the order of 95%. (Seriously.) Not only have I spared myself enormous effort but I have effectively neutralised a whole raft of potentially esteem-crushing disappointments. Sure, I still get caught out, and on occasion I elect to play the 'all round fabulous guy' card, but the liberating effect has been pronounced. If you do only one thing on this list – do this. Walk away from the mirror.

It does take practise but, if someone as deeply vain as me can manage it, I'm fairly sure you can.

9: Drill down into desire – what is it you truly want?

Thus far we have talked a lot about behavior; now it's time to address desire. Getting clear about our desires is a massively liberating form of awareness. In saying this I am *not* suggesting that you rush out and sign up to one of the numerous puritanical programmes aimed at delegitimising, controlling and/or denying desire, but rather that you try to understand it. More accurately identify it.

What actually is it you desire?

Let me frame it another way: when you say that you want a fancy, expensive new car is it really the object or the feeling you believe the getting of the object will deliver? Why indeed do we want success or wealth – is it the cash or the feeling its accumulation engenders? With the exception of practical survival-based wishes like the desire for predictable access to food and shelter, or handy tools that save labour and increase efficiency, most of our deeper, longer term desires revolve around the triggering of pleasing feeling states. Or, if you prefer it more neuro-scientific, the activation of reward centres in the brain. It's the 'feeling good' that we're chasing, not the circular bit of metal hanging on the end of a colourful ribbon.

In effect, once we begin to untangle the nexus between the place-holding objects of our desire (Oscars, firmer thighs, another tattoo, etc) and the psycho-emotional rewards attached to them, we can gain a bigger picture perspective on ourselves and our wants, dreams and ambitions. This, in turn, creates a moment of pause and reflection – is the pursuit of this goal really worth it? Can I get the same feeling from something else? In fact, *why* do I want this feeling? Or even, do I *really* want this feeling, or … ?

As a bare minimum this kind of questioning gives us room to stop, take a deep breath and re-evaluate; and this goes a long way to identifying and disempowering external narratives and unconscious internal habits. Then, if you get good at it, you can defuse all manner of wish-fulfilment fantasy and striving mantras and bring more of your attention and energy back from an imagined future – when desire will supposedly be sated – and into a more grateful present where those pleasing feeling states are happening right now.

Because it may well be that, if you switch your focus, you will discover that you already have what you want.

10: Do the same with fear – and then ask honestly if your fears are reasonable?

Firstly, let's be honest, *some* fears are well-grounded. Furthermore, fear is a brilliantly effective evolutionary adaptation. Don't let the spiritual truth warriors and other ideologues fool you into pathologising all your fears.

Our challenge then is to work out which of our fears represent prudent caution and which are indicative of a debilitating paranoia or a symptom of unnecessary drama. Upon examination, most will likely reveal themselves to be either unfounded or, as in the case of aging and death, futile. Indeed, even a quarter-reasonable risk analysis will reveal that the odds of being killed by terrorists or eaten by a shark are pretty slim. The media may well be a gaudy spectacle of death and dread but you don't need to a be Mensa member to know that this is driven by a desire to exploit us all in order to shift units and, further, to psychologically manipulate us into this or that way of thinking. Quite simply, the nightly news, the internet and the idiotic circus of modern democracy are not reliable guides to the true measure of real danger in the world.

On a more personal scale, fears around loneliness, unpopularity, abandonment and so on are also worth unpacking. Do they contribute to my overall well-being? How do they manifest in my relationships with others and myself? Do they impel me towards ultimately poor decision making? In fact, are my fears simply habits of thinking? Did I just copy them from my parents? And anyway, whose fear *is* this?

Fear, like desire, when looked at calmly, often dissolves. And even if it doesn't, teasing it apart will help to keep it in perspective and allow you the space to consider alternative strategies and behaviours.

11: Observe and coolly assess your progress – give rewards and outline further questions and challenges.

Like any long term project, trying to distinguish your truest inner voice and authentic self from the morass of noise in your head will involve a trial and error journey. In this particular instance it is a process which may never end and where the very definitions of end point and success are vague. That said, the results will begin to flow well before any nominated finish line and – in all but the most bizarre and unforeseeable circumstances – quite likely prior to conclusive events like death, coma or dementia.

In order to properly monitor outcomes and maintain motivation, it pays to pay attention. (Indeed, this entire project is really one of awareness and attention. This is just another opportunity for you to practise the skills and discipline required.) However, it is vital not simply to recognise and penalise failure but to acknowledge and honour success. Allow yourself rewards for the positives and use the setbacks as a cue to hone your Q&A dialogue and set fresh challenges.

This is about working towards a sustainable balance between compassionate encouragement and fearless honesty. It takes practise, of course, but as with the list items above, the act of practising is in itself part of the overall process.

From my own experience, I can report that as time went by this became easier, less deliberate and more intuitive. In essence what was happening was that I was tuning in more frequently and with increasing clarity to the core truths of my life and identity. In other words, I was distilling my authentic self from the slurry and finding it ever easier to think, feel and act in accordance with my own, genuinely self-authored beliefs and objectives.

12: Practise enjoying the little things.

I know, you've heard it a million times. The 'gratitude thing' gets a mention in almost every self-help, pop-shrinkery tract and life coaching manual out there. However, don't let the Oprahfication of gratitude put you off, because training yourself to take pleasure and be thankful for the little things is as near to profound and life altering as it gets for most of us. In a culture addicted to the grand, the mighty and the perfectly sexy, the joy to be had in the aroma of good coffee or the feel of freshly laundered sheets is too often overlooked.

Okay, so we know this but …

As with much of the above, the trick is to practise the focus required to transport gratitude from Facebook meme to daily reality. So, those little rewards I just mentioned in point 11 – how about starting off with them?

Viewed through a risk/reward prism, thankfulness is a stunningly good investment. The dividends are frequent and manifold. I won't bore you by listing them but I will say that gratitude, like so much in our lives, is a habit. Indeed, it's a gateway drug to liberation and happiness; and I'll be honest, I'm hooked.

Sure, it may seem a tad lame and 'latte set' but, in your own time and your own way, you will almost certainly reap substantial benefits from the enjoyment of little things. (As examples, my personal faves include the aquatint light in the beachside suburb where I live, the chatter of birds, discovering a cool new tune and the sheer ecstasy of fresh bread and butter. Nothing too grandiose about any of that, is there?)

13: Practise letting the small shit go – identify what you can and cannot control – pick your battles.

Like gratitude, this one is widely touted. *Don't sweat the small shit.* Aside from any putatively spiritual benefits this one's very practical. Given that you've only got a certain amount of energy and attention, why tie so much of it up stressing about what bitchface thinks? After all, time is ticking by.

The key change agents here are our old friends awareness and practise – interrupting old habits and laying down new ones. If you find yourself stuck in a cycle of angst over something, find a moment to ask yourself how important this will seem in five years. Often, zooming out from a storm of stress, anger or disappointment reveals all too clearly its relative insignificance. Indeed, most of the things we get het up about are tiny dramas. Not much more than hissy-fits.

In addition, most of us, at some point, get massively confused about what we can and can't control. Reminding ourselves that our domain is actually quite limited (although far from insignificant) is pivotal to the practise of letting shit go. Despite all those slave narratives out there, our kingdom is ourselves – our responses, our behaviours, where we put our focus, what we spend our time on, etc. Consciously identifying the scope of our control and remembering this in moments of tension creates an extremely useful valve of stress relief and sets up the conditions for divorcing the drama; quite apart from allowing you to cross a whole bunch of crap off the work load.

So just start. Pick something small and relatively easy to begin with. Something you normally find yourself getting tight over but which, intellectually, you know is pretty trivial. (Some little OCD thing you do.) After a while, as you begin to establish and expand this new strategy of letting go, you may well, as I did, begin to reap the surprising and beautiful reward of lightness. Letting stuff drop is a form of psycho-emotional weight loss you can sense mentally and physically. Even though you might not be able to measure it on the scales you will almost certainly *feel* lighter. Having less to worry about is a blessed relief and, in turn, leaves you with more energy for the stuff that *really* matters to you.

14: Practise experimenting with external change – try stuff, see how it goes – be playful with it sometimes.

The trouble with most self-improvement ideologies and enlightenment projects is that they're no fun. Indeed, most are framed in censorious and punishing terms and, although they won't admit it, they usually want you to deny yourself pleasure, (especially sensual pleasure). What's more, because they mandate end points, they are narrow and reductionist and quash improvisation and experiment.

However, since our goal with this '15 things thing' is simply to identify and be in contact with a truer inner voice – without the fascist control of better, wiser, purer objectives – we can tinker, have fun with it, try stuff out. So, when you think you're starting to get clearer signals from the channel of the real you, start doing the stuff it suggests. Initially, this may involve a greater percentage of 'not doing that shit anymore' but as you begin to enjoy the rewards of quitting you will find new behaviours, new routines, to replace those dreary old obedience rituals. Sure, some will be dead ends. So what, try something else next time. Remember: *it doesn't matter in the end!*

Also, there is no legislated *amount* of change required. You don't have to be drastic – although you most certainly can be. It's not like you need to ditch your job in town and move to a co-operatively managed eco-village, or indeed become celibate, polyamorous, teetotal or 5000% organic. The idea, after all, is to practise and refine methods for doing whatever *you* want.

15: Frame any choices and changes in risk/reward terms – dilute unrealistic, utopian expectations and disempower dystopian fear narratives.

Finally, to return to one of the core tenets of the book, practise viewing the entire process and the attendant results through a cost/benefit prism. Accept and understand that with reward comes cost. With gains, losses. All choice involves risk. The world contains uncertainties and unknowables. Utopias and dystopias are infantile, linear control fantasies. Simplistic, unrealistic and ultimately self-defeating recipes for disappointment, punishment and continued slavery. Fuck that shit.

In contrast, the existential/economic mindset I have discussed throughout encourages risk and innovation by factoring in the likelihood of so called failure and by stripping out both punitive judgement and hubristic excess. It demythologises both process and outcome. Removes all must imperatives. It simply hands you a bunch of temporal capital (time, life dollars, etc) and lets you spend it where you may.

Without the weight of Essentialist meaning baggage and the right/wrong dichotomies it imposes, you are free to invest in a portfolio of belief, behaviour, lifestyle and relationships, and to shift the weighting of your investment in accordance with both current and predicted market conditions. To go with the flow, tweak, re-position, re-calibrate, fuck up totally and bounce right back. To play the free market of life and identity. To choose the voice you speak with – to others and, more importantly, to yourself.

In my experience, having tried all the above and more, I have found that the voice of the 'authentic me' is something like a guide, a kindly professor or therapist. It has yet to be badly wrong (in slight error sometimes maybe but not disastrously so) and is never nailed into ideology or assertive certainty. It never pulls rank and does not insist that I just take its word for it. It is not a boss or final authority, neither is it a flatterer or excuse maker. Indeed, it never gives orders, it simply suggests. It offers me a choice and leaves me to take what course of action I may.

Beneath all the particulars though what jumps out is that we can, with effort, focus and discipline, change the way we speak to ourselves and, in the process, tag and filter out noise that we have simply internalised. Just as we need not be the slaves of external signals, so too we are not bound to be the victims of our own internal haranguing. Our fears, our persecution complexes, the reflexive hankering for herd approval – all of these can be challenged and their power to drive habitual behaviour revoked.

It may well be that you already have your own methods, or will evolve entirely different strategies, but I feel confident that if you can clearly identify your own true beliefs and objectives and distinguish them from the welter of received tropes, imperatives and value judgements, you will significantly increase the likelihood of sustainable happiness going forward. Which is I why I wrote this book and, I'm guessing, why you chose to read it.

Good luck. ☺

BONUS MATERIAL

Although the ten chapters of the book proper have endeavoured to set out a step-by-step case, it would be dishonest of me to pretend that the guts of everything I've argued isn't somehow rooted in deeply personal experiences and narratives. So here I conclude on a more autobiographical note; if only to further underline the notion that all these fine philosophical ideas and bold assertions serve a core psycho-emotional purpose and stem from a highly idiosyncratic perspective. Thus, if you're looking to put a little more (human) flesh on the bones of *The Pointless Revolution*, read Appendices 2 and 3.

PS: If however you're more interested in the teasing out of ideas related to but slightly tangential to the main arguments of the book, read the *(Not Quite) Random Yet (Kinda) Relevant Other Bits* section starting on the page opposite.

APPENDIX 1.
{NOT QUITE} RANDOM YET {KINDA} RELEVANT OTHER BITS

or

The bits that didn't quite fit in elsewhere

It's as though we have been beating a kind of retreat from what we truly are. And hey presto: squeaky clean air-conditioned condos, gated communities and digital atomisation. Not to mention the bewildering idiocy of presidentially promised border walls and the freakishly immobile spectacle of Botox faces and silicon tits. It's like King Canute on steroids!

In this Appendix I have strung together a few short observations and musings that cluster around our central themes.

These are the side dishes that didn't quite make it onto the main menu but which, I feel, expand and consolidate a few key points. These, in order, are:

- The 'nature' problem
- The mono-causal fallacy
- The failure of conspiracy
- The blame/shame game

THE 'NATURE' PROBLEM

Perhaps our key problem with nature is the word itself; or rather, what its use as a catch-all term for anything in the world that isn't either human or 'man made' signifies.

Though our English word 'nature' has its roots in the Latin 'natura' (meaning essential quality or innate disposition), which in turn has echoes in 'natal' (as in 'birth'), our application of the word to delineate the rest of the environment from ourselves is indicative of a fundamental schism. The manner in which we use and generally understand terms like *the natural world*, *Mother Nature* and *natural healing* casts nature as the other. As an externality. There's us, the humans, and then there's *it*, nature. This so-called nature includes everything else in the biosphere, plus all aspects of weather, geology, glacial oscillation, plate tectonics, lunar activity and, since Darwin, the ongoing process of evolution itself. Some of us probably include the rest of the cosmos in the nature basket. Point is, in our common conceptualisation, nature – or environment – lives outside us.

In one way, of course, this is no big deal; just a banal result of the basic I/Not I dichotomy. Furthermore, as a social species we were always going to group identify in Us/Not Us terms. You might even say it's only natural. Yet, when we look around us, it's not hard to see how we humans are living in a fashion that jeopardises our survival within the planetary biosphere that sustains us. In addition, we have come to regard nature as both a larder and a general commodity for our exploitation. As property. Indeed, since the Agricultural Revolution profoundly shifted the dynamics of food supply, our relationship with nature has been based on dominance. *We* are the masters, the owners, and we have a bunch of gods, tools and deeds of title to back us up on that. Little wonder our current economic, political and cultural orthodoxies continue to generate the kind of unsustainable resource use, atmospheric and oceanic pollution, and subsequent biodiversity loss that seems increasingly likely to bring our species to an existential crunch point.

Would such a trajectory even be possible if we genuinely – not just in a dry, intellectual fashion but in a deeply intuitive, attitudinal way – regarded ourselves as *part* of nature? *In* nature? As animals, just like we regard antelopes, fish and owls? As natural phenomena, like trees, clouds and mountains? Bit part players in a symbiotic, synergistic unfolding? What if we didn't even recognise the Human/Nature distinction?

Not for one moment am I suggesting that our disconnect from nature explains all our cruelties and follies, nor indeed that a re-connection will magically cure all our ills. However, I am suggesting that by extracting ourselves from the environment we evolved in, and are adapted to, we concurrently laid the foundations for both the individual psycho-emotional and broader herd-think conditions required for the development of abstract societies, and the denialist cultures we find ourselves in now. We wouldn't live the way we live, and maybe wouldn't even have an 'environment issue' if we didn't fundamentally regard ourselves as somehow outside of nature and specifically excluded from its finely tuned balance.

Whereas the promulgators of middle class guilt would like us to believe that capitalism and Western society is the cause, it is plain that our separation from nature pre-dates modern consumerism by thousands, if not tens of thousands of years. In fact, what we see in many ancient cultures and cosmologies is the personification and deification of nature, where the wider world is cast as the other and our relationship to it rooted firmly in servitude and fear. For most of human history we have lived in the thrall of nature's uncertainties – would it rain, etc – as well as its inevitabilities; principally disease and death. Given this, it is no surprise that our forebears strove to tame a world that always seemed to threaten them with extinction, using everything from prayer and ritual sacrifice to spears and skins. For all our self-righteous hindsight we can hardly blame our ancestors for wanting to survive, just like we can't reasonably criticise birds for building nests or lambaste penguins for hanging out in huge huddles when it gets too cold.

However, unlike koalas or leopards, we evolved the brain power to elevate and energise our survival strategies to the point where caution and justifiable fear morphed into control and dominion. As an apex predator we out-flanked the other animals, adapted to and planned for a broader range of environmental contingencies and, with language, were able to codify and transmit accrued knowledge and practise in a much more precise way. With time we were able to put an ever increasing gap between ourselves and the things that threatened to eat, freeze and invade us. Then, when we invented agriculture, we started to believe that even starvation could be held at bay. That we could *always* have food.

Nature 0, Humanity 1.

Unfortunately for our early farming forebears, grain surpluses did nothing to mitigate the certainty of death. Nor did bulging granaries and complex social organisation do much to prevent plagues, droughts and earthquakes. In fact, not even the gods seemed prepared to step in and prevent us ageing and dying – notwithstanding that we slit the throats of bulls and sometimes murdered virgins to show them how serious we were about this 'not wanting to get sick and die' stuff. Dammit, that pesky nature just wouldn't go away.

Still, we kept on trying and eventually we concocted a way of living that was so sanitised, so removed from seasonal fluctuations that we were able to externalise nature as a mere photo opportunity. A news spectacle (cyclone, tsunami, heat wave) or a nice family friendly wildlife documentary. Nature is something we watch, rather than participate in. We go camping in it. We 'get back' to it. Either that, or consume it – mine it, harvest it, catch it, kill it. And now of course we're actively tweaking it, fiddling with the DNA of plants, people and other animals in an attempt to render nature entirely in the fashion of our own liking.

So what, you might think. Isn't this just evolution at work?

My word it is. In fact, that's part of the point I'm trying to make. If humanity gets so smart that we undo ourselves with our cleverness, then evolution will have seen off yet another species. If, in trying to immortalise ourselves, we create the conditions for own demise, so be it. The central denial, and the manifold avoidance strategies it has fuelled, will have directly contributed to bringing about the very thing it was most scared of. (Irony much?)

In saying this I am not contending that civilisation collapse and/or species extinction is inevitable. Likewise, I am not arguing for a return to living on the savannah in small clan groups subsisting on root vegetables and running away from lions. Apocalypse and utopia are both simplistic narratives, so let's leave them to the bourgeois hairshirts and other fundamentalist droners.

Rather, I am pointing at both the hubris and denial (fear) that operates in our collective cultural subconscious, and also at the more obviously manifest mechanisms of command and control that we see across every ethnicity, in all religions and every political and economic system, as well as up and down the class and wealth ladder. In fact, everywhere in human societies. Moreover, what I'm suggesting is that our ingrained us/it view of nature is no longer serving us (or it, for that matter). Aside from collectively creating dead zones in the ocean and sowing the seeds of potentially catastrophic methane release from melting permafrost, when I look around me I see people everywhere on mad individual crusades to purchase this, achieve that, be sexier and do, climb or listen to the 1001 compulsory whatever the fuck. Maybe none of this would concern me – and I wouldn't be writing this book – if it felt like we were all happy doing this.

Drilling right into the core, it strikes me that our relationship 'with' nature (as if it were somehow something other) is akin to our relationship with one another and, perhaps even more salient, ourselves. It's not just that a foundational separation – I/Not I – is required for identity consciousness to arise and for you and I to experience what we call a *life*, it's that once the distinction is made the I, like every other complex system in the universe, is in the persistence business. It's just that in our case the I knows that it will one day cease to be I; will merge back into the Not I. Into nature. This central awareness and the resulting fear of unbeing have driven us to more clearly define and 'thicken up' the border zone between life and death, between us and nature. Between each other. It's as though we have been beating a kind of retreat from what we truly are. And hey presto: squeaky clean air-conditioned condos, gated communities and digital atomisation. Not to mention the bewildering idiocy of presidentially-promised border walls and the freakishly immobile spectacle of Botox faces and silicon tits. It's like King Canute on steroids!

For it's one thing to make prudent plans and execute clever strategies to survive, it's another to create a form of survival mired in self-defeating fear and suicidal arrogance. After all, mortal terror is ultimately futile, and even the most pridefully constructed and complex systems of defence will yield to the unravelling of time and entropy.

Thus, the term 'nature' should be an almost meaningless banality, synonymous with 'universe' and 'existence'. Everything is in nature … even you. Even these keystrokes.

THE MONO-CAUSAL FALLACY

All the while I was composing and editing the previous section I was on guard, eager not to drift into the wildly popular but seriously dumbed down domain of the single cause theory.

This is the commonplace mode of thinking which suggests that Outcome X is wholly caused by Antecedent Y. Whilst this mechanism works neatly in children's storybooks and Hollywood blockbusters it is, in my view, grossly inadequate as a serious explanation for complex phenomena such as occur in the multi-faceted, deeply entangled world of reality. So, rather than suggesting that our disconnect from nature is the *sole cause* of this ill and that malady, what I'm contending is that it is a big *contributing factor*, one of a number of inputs into the causation equation that has led us here.

Now this might seem super fucking obvious – and I mean, really, it is; or at least it damn well should be – yet the mono-causal fallacy not only persists but appears to be the norm. Facebook feeds and tabloid news bulletins are full of it. Modern democracy deals it out like so much baby food; mushed up goo for infant electors. Marketing mavens and ad creatives cynically exploit our penchant for one stop analysis. *Keep it simple, stupid*, they proudly declare. Even so-called 'alternative' types dish out simplistic, catchphrase explanations, blaming the patriarchy, PC or the 1% for just about everything. The ubiquity of sound bite culture and our evident weakness for ethnic, gender and generational stereotypes further illustrate our tendency to take the instant fix answer and run with it. (We can see how the current wave of so-called identity politics stems from and amplifies this tendency.)

Like the 'narrative palliative' I discussed back in Chapter 4, the mono-causal fallacy suggests an infantile (at best juvenile) predisposition. In its own way it is an attempt to transfigure a complex, uncertain world into a simpler, safer and far more predictable place, where one thing neatly follows another in a basic linear relationship. Or, for the conspiracists and entitlement paranoiacs out there, it makes the world seem entirely poisonous and vexatious, thereby feeding into their victim psychodrama of *it's not fair, told you so, they're out to get me*.

In a way the mono-causal fallacy is not so far removed from our erstwhile faith in ancient gods, it rained because we prayed real well and the crops only grew because we ritually raped and murdered those young girls back in the spring. Okay, so the example is extreme but the point is that our susceptibility to blunt 'X makes Y happen' cause and effect arguments remains largely in place. Religious and political extremists understand this only too well, which is why they constantly pitch to it.

However, aside from ensuring that the cultural and political airwaves hum along to a soundtrack of relentless stupidity, the mono-cause mindset plays out in homes and workplaces. It fuels our love of simple, band-aid solutions and the subsequent disappointment and frustration we feel when the evidence contradicts our previous assertions. Sometimes called cognitive dissonance, this is the discomfort that springs from actions and information that impel us to question or confront our beliefs and values. It is, it seems, often too much for many of us. The 'silo' phenomenon – our preference for self-reflecting channels of information – illustrates this all too well. If reality proves too grey and nuanced, too difficult, we retreat into a ring-fenced fortress of amplified agreement. Whilst this may also be said of those who profess *not* to have crude black/white views, the dissonance cost is higher for the mono-causals, if only because the simpler the belief the more fervently it tends to be held. Letting go of mildly held opinions is far easier than the dislocating jolt of re-appraising strongly held articles of faith. After all, it's passionate believers who flee to bunkers and cult compounds, let alone strap on suicide vests.

On a cost/benefit basis, mono-cause thinking strikes me as a very poor investment. Though there is the upfront sugar hit of surety, and the effort saving expedience of a quick and easy decision, the risk of being contradicted by reality is so high – pretty well inevitable really – that the ongoing dividends seem more likely to be confusion and disappointment, or maybe frustration, blame and anger. Perhaps even an overriding sense that 'things are going down the tube'. Or more dangerously, outright fear and its scowling sidekick: hate.

Unfortunately for those of us of who understand that the world is an extraordinarily complex network of sometimes competing, sometimes coalescing, always changing forces, and that life does not unfold like cute little stories do, we are surrounded by people who either can't or won't accept this. Their prejudices, paranoias and poorly thought through actions and opinions affect us. Our key psycho-emotional challenge, ironically, is not to let these ideologues and idiots drive us towards our own versions of mono-causality; namely, we are in this parlous position because most people are fuckwits. Indeed, it behoves us to remember that even though selfishness, tribalism, ideological fantasy and childlike thinking have certainly contributed to the shape of things, so too have a huge number of other inputs – including the mechanics of power, the urgencies of economy and a myriad of historic, technological and personal circumstances. Y'know, and the small matter of evolution.

So, whilst the mono-causal fallacy *is* a problem, it's not the sole cause of:

- (Insert favourite socio-cultural blight.)

I bother to mention this because, to be honest, I *am* currently (circa 2019) experiencing a form of misanthropic disgust response to the prevailing culture of myopic idiocy and intellectual laziness that seems to surround me and, therefore, am taking this opportunity to remind myself *not* to slide into hermetic bitterness – not because being a loner is inherently bad but because I sense that the principal dividends of attaching too strongly to a *humanity is totally fucked* belief will be unhappiness and mistrust. Thus, while I'm fine for you to call me a snob or an elitist, I'm not so keen on a life of grumpy and suspicious isolation.

Instead, in the existential/economic spirit of this book, I am preferencing and practising the rigour and discipline of being critical, rather than getting swept up in the righteous drama of outrage. (There *is* a difference.) And anyway, I wouldn't wanna lurch into conspiratorial victim mania. I mean, *that* sounds truly awful.

THE FAILURE OF CONSPIRACY

Quick, drop everything (except your guns). Retire to the nearest awakened, organic bunker. The Asian, Muslim, central banking, lizard controlled, patriarchal lesbian cyborgs are just about to put their multi-thousand year action plan into overdrive. They've read every word in this book, and they listened in while you were reading it, and they're prepping up chemtrails and vaccine shots in covert Rothschild financed water treatment plants situated beneath the Vatican, while their puppet PC politicians prepare to destroy parents' rights and make it illegal to have a penis. Oh no — only the internet can save us now!*

(* Except that the internet is also a tool of data mining oppression designed to disseminate ridiculous conspiracy theories in order to distract you from what's REALLY going on.)

Clearly, the life of the conspiracist is one of remorseless, dystopian oppression. They look out at the world and see a vale of poison. If penis wielding patriarchs aren't systematically raping you with phallus shaped shards of the nearest glass ceiling, vagina toting ninja feminists are hiding around every corner ready to confiscate your cock and scramble your gender identity. Every time it rains evil chemicals designed to pacify you or render you infertile are leeching into your bloodstream. Illuminati agents disguised as doctors, nurses and aid workers are trawling health clinics, schools and squalid refugee camps giving innocent little kiddies injections designed to make them autistic. Next up, it's Shari'a law and compulsory Mandarin classes. Then, to make matters worse, there's a permanently looming apocalypse to contend with.

On the plus side though, there's the smug satisfaction of being one of the awakened elite, of being in the vanguard of the new dawn, of heralding the great paradigm shift. Kinda like those kids who blow up other kids at pop concerts. Y'know, really taking a stand against oppression. Paving the way for the Mahdi and all that.

All jokes aside, the conspiracy mantra is one of the most loudly proclaimed and seductive slave narratives out there. It is textbook victim thinking; but hyped up into super-charged paranoia by a combination of lazy conflation, false equivalence, selective amnesia, mono-causal mania and, let's be frank, a crudely reductionist and dehumanising view of the enemy of choice. These people think they're *sooo* alternative and yet their apparent analysis is rooted in exactly the same kind of monochromatic essentialisation we associate with McCarthyist 'red scares' and post-911 Islamophobia. Their enemy is always working covertly, employing invisible hands at every level for nefarious ends. In addition, whilst castigating the mainstream media for its blatant fear mongering, conspiracists use the very same lures to get our attention – impending catastrophe, heinous villainy, simplistic narrative. Like ideologically driven zealots throughout history, conspiracy junkies resort to emotive propaganda.

However, let's be fair, underneath their overblown hysteria and righteous slavethink, these folks are quite right to call into question the mechanisms of the power complex, and to highlight the distorting effects of entrenched privilege and the undue influence of extreme wealth. Indeed, as I have noted many times previously, there is still plenty of injustice, prejudice, barefaced dishonesty, wanton disregard and even outright Machiavellian cynicism embedded in our economy, polity and more broadly across our societies. Furthermore, there is undoubtedly collusion and conniving aplenty, with secret deals and all the rest of it. Then there are the brain crushingly dumb control narratives of religion and the lobotomised spectacles of contemporary Western democracy and celebrity worship.

So yes, it's true, there *are* those who seek to control and exploit. Some of them are in power or sit on highly remunerated boards – but so too some are your friends, your parents, your spouse. Some may even be your kids. In fact, most of us have pulled this kinda shit at one time or another. I know I have.

The point here is that *humans* act in competitive, self-interested ways. (Not just white men or Jewish banking families, but all of us.) We seek specific advantage for ourselves and whatever in-group we feel part of. Once we have something we want to keep it, whether its power, territory, prestige or cash. Meanwhile, others may try to take it from us. Sometimes they'll use violence and coercion, other times argument and moral pressure. They may even resort to lies, bribery and subterfuge. However, blinded by the drama of their own fundamentalism, our conspiracy cousins have reduced the multi-variate complexity of individual and herd behaviour to an infantile storybook narrative, where people and individual responsibility are airbrushed out and mechanistic, centrally organised inevitability is wheeled in to replace it. If Disney did dystopia, this would be their cartoon *1984*. (Perhaps they could call the book tie-in *Orwellian Hell For Dummies*. That'd sell.)

Okay, so let's run through three of the fundamental gaps in the conspiracy case, because, aside from narrative reduction there are a number of glaring holes in their much cherished vision of totalitarian oppression.

1: Is such a conspiracy even necessary?

One of the central tenets of most conspiracy theories is that whichever secretive cabal supposedly rules us, it works assiduously to keep us stupid, selfish, myopic, competitive and distracted. The obvious question is, would you even *need* a conspiracy for that?

No disrespect folks – but, seriously? Where is the evidence that it would *require* a bunch of evil-doers to *concoct* the conditions for these things to exist and flourish? Selfishness, tribalism, nimbyism*, short term narrow focus, greed, prejudice and simplistic thinking are long established and commonplace human traits. As indeed is our evolved tendency for hierarchical social structures. It didn't require an agricultural or industrial revolution to entrench the basic dynamics of power or to establish rules governing individual behaviour in the herd context. As for 'distracted', let's face it, most of us are not overly interested in the abstractions, complexities and the minutiae of politics and power, so long as we feel able to conduct our private, family and communal lives with minimum (tolerable) levels of interference, a good amount of readily accessible social services and reliable protection from random predation. In fact, we are quite happy to delegate the difficult headache of governing to others because we'd rather just live happy lives with those we love. (Which is a perfectly okay thing to want.)

The fact that our twenty-first century model of bread and circuses is a 24/7, multi-channel onslaught of pantomime, mob-amusing idiocy is a) hardly surprising; and b) says at least as much about the supposedly noble 99% as it ever has about the apparently nasty 1%. Indeed, to cast the populace as somehow innocent in this mix is more than just an absurd ideological us/them fantasy, it's a full blown cop out.

(* Nimbyism: the 'not in my back yard' phenomenon.)

2: **Would such a conspiracy succeed?**

The standard conspiracy model has it that there is a developed and detailed plan for the deliberate and ongoing manipulation of every aspect of economy, polity, history and culture for the primary benefit of a tiny cadre – whatever form it might take.

In order to succeed as a covert and totalitarian operation such a plan would require not only 100% agreement and superbly seamless co-operation and execution from said conspirators but – because the theory also goes that this is a *repressive* complex – a not inconsiderable enforcement apparatus and an effective propaganda arm. All of which means people. Party members, employees, consultants, hired goons, etc. On paper and screen – in novels, films and on numerous websites – this appears doable. However, the theoretical edifice of conspiracy reckons without the flawed input of *actual human beings*. Y'know, those fractious, covetous, error prone, forgetful, lazy and impetuous creatures. Folks like us.

However, it's not just regulation human frailty that the conspirators have to contend with. The sheer scale and nature of their cunning plan creates two obvious and empire shattering risks.

Firstly, given the enormity and complexity of the task, our small band of Big Brothers would need to co-opt an army of competent sidekicks, thereby creating the 'problem of the palace guard'. Basically, our shadowy rulers would need to take on the enormous risk of creating and empowering the very force most likely to expose and/or overthrow them. For along with the huge organisational burden that furtively ruling the world entails comes a fair sized workforce; people in enough of the know to blow the whole thing to smithereens. A cursory glance at history furnishes us with countless examples of palace coups, from the Praetorian Guard's frequent toppling and murder of Roman emperors to the litany of military takeovers that have ousted kings, presidents and PMs across the millennia. Indeed, most revolutions are inside jobs.

Secondly, the hugely secret nature of their plan automatically creates a massive incentive for bean-spilling, which in turn generates opportunities for blackmailing co-conspirators and for playing the heroic whistle-blower. To suppose that our conniving overlords, or indeed any of their numerous lieutenants, would somehow always remain beyond such petty temptation is to dehumanise them, to ascribe to them a machine like quality of adherence; or perversely, to make them slaves to their own power. (Uneasy rests the head that wears the crown and all that.)

So, whilst we may not be able to say with *absolute certainty* that no centrally organised and currently functioning coalition of global control exists, we can say that the probability, given the necessary participation of human beings, is extremely remote.

What's more, if this wicked conspiracy *is* afoot it has already manifestly failed on the secrecy score. I mean, just about every bunker-stocking, pseudo-rebellious, paranoid slave on the internet appears to have unmasked the key villains and, what's more, posted a meme to that effect. In fact, don't we already know that everything we've been told is a lie?

3: Would such a conspiracy of dominion ever be seriously embarked upon?

Let's suppose we wanted to get together and hatch a plan for global domination, our principal motives being those old staples wealth and power. At some point, if we were sane and thinking things through properly (doing our due diligence), the question would be asked: *given that our goal is wealth and power, what's the best way for us to achieve that objective and, furthermore, to ensure the continuation of our privilege into the foreseeable future?*

Perhaps at first we would opt for brute force and theft. However, we would soon discover that violence, coercion and the greedy hoarding of all the best goodies automatically creates passionate opposition, or at the very least widespread resentment and mistrust. So now we need troops to help us fend off the disgruntled mob. This will be both expensive and dangerous, because now we've trained and armed a force that could just as easily bribe us for a bigger share of the spoils or maybe even kill us in our beds. Turns out that the sword thing, (live by/die by), is true after all – and so now we've effectively condemned ourselves to a huge wage bill, an endless organisational headache and a fortress lifestyle of constant wariness; if not permanent and debilitating paranoia. Power underwritten by forceful suppression is costly, time consuming and ultimately defeats its own purpose.

Again, assuming sanity and an ability to see beyond the next five minutes, we would eventually work out that the most sustainable power model involved a level of sharing out both the costs and the benefits of empire. In addition, we would soon figure out that the creation and imposition of a control architecture that fostered a low-trust society would effectively 'bake in' the conditions for a risk-averse, potentially stagnant economy and, furthermore, a calcification of the socio-cultural space and the loss of creativity and adaptability this would entail.

Whilst some will argue that this is exactly where humanity finds itself right now, it is another to suppose that this state of affairs arose because a few sinister folk planned things with precisely this outcome in mind. If indeed we are in a 'parlous state' it is most likely the result of multiple/incremental follies and honest errors, as opposed to being the neatly sculpted by-product of an act of centrally organised and sustained suicidal insanity. The fear-based, poison world society of the shadowy overlord is hardly a great pay-off for all that tiring conspiring and the ever-present fear of exposure and palace rebellion. After all, where's the fun in spending every minute micro-managing the exhaustive detail and tracking the finances of an oppressive power complex? *I mean, c'mon, when do we get to snort this top shelf coke from the tanned midriffs of the sexy young things we've lured onto our yacht?*

In fact, the more we think about it the more ill-advised our investment in this world domination biz seems.

So instead, let's just say that in order to keep the mob pacified we agree to devolve some of our considerable power to others – even if we're still pretty keen on the untold wealth idea. Trouble is, as we now know, an oppressive apparatus and the belief that everything is kinda rigged create moribund social and economic conditions. Fear, mistrust and the orthodoxy they engender don't tend to favour entrepreneurial spirit, bold innovation and wealth generating risk. Rather than relying on our clique of 'world rulers' to come up with *every single* good idea and/or become the default universal wage payer, we would soon discover that there's far more profit and sustainable growth to be had for much less effort in a dynamic, diversified economy; one in which people feel they have incentives other than the mere avoidance of expensively assembled death squads.

By now I'm sure you can see where this is heading. If, as conspiracy ideologues insist, there is a fixed and central cabal that 'rules the world' according to an agreed plan, then, provided these central banking reptiles are even vaguely sensible and self-regarding (let alone historically and economically literate), their best option would be an open, pluralistic, trust-based society with a flexible, dynamic economy that required the least amount of violent enforcement and a minimum of deal-breaking secrets.

Thus, if we *were* to gather in some gilded palace to devise a solid, ongoing means of divvying up the world between us, we would ultimately conclude that, on a risk/reward basis, a broad based peaceable freedom would be the most reliable and least onerous way of generating lasting wealth and privilege for ourselves. We would work out that to enslave others is to enslave ourselves. And what would be the fucking point of that?

Considering the various probabilities and factoring in the flawed humanity of the participants, an insane and completely unnecessary conspiracy doomed to almost certain failure seems to be something that only an intellectual minnow and/or psychopath with virtually no self-awareness or psycho-emotional savvy would even contemplate.

Again, being fair, absurdly unlikely as it seems, the global dystopia beloved of conspiracy zealots is not technically impossible. Like you and I, power elites will act in their own perceived interest. Looking around, it's plain to see evidence of this and, as many economic analysts have found, global wealth disparity has increased significantly since 1980, with social and financial inequality returning to pre-WW1 levels*. Clearly, many of those with power and influence have and will continue to feather their own nests, often at the expense of others. Our societies are, as they have invariably been for millennia, deeply hierarchical, and many structural injustices remain firmly in place. Though this is undesirable, unfair and unjust we cannot honestly pretend that this is either a recent invention, the sole responsibility of a narrowly defined group or, indeed, all that astonishing.

(* Most notably the French economist Thomas Piketty, whose 2013 book *Capital In The Twenty-First Century* details this claim.)

In the end, my bottom line issue with the conspiracy narrative is not so much its fantastical over-read and dehumanising prejudices, it's that, as a critique of power, it is counter-productive. Easily dismissed on account of its simplistic conceptualisation and moralising undergraduate tone, it de-legitimises its own agenda, making genuine analysis and activism easier to pigeon hole. In effect, conspiracy theorists prop up the status quo with their use of textbook propaganda techniques and their tabloid appeal to basic us/them, good/evil dichotomies, which then help to further dumb down and polemicise the discourse. The tropes of conspiracy are simply another version of the blame culture, another form of crude identity politics, another way of insisting upon an orthodox view. I suspect that many of our comrades in the dystopia scene would make exemplary Stalinist tyrants.

Luckily for the rest of us, conspiracy fans are generally lazy fundamentalists. For all their hardcore ideological angst they mostly lack the backbone to get off You Tube and do anything to make a better world for their fellow human beings – let alone set up a puritanically rigid dystopia of their own.

THE BLAME / SHAME GAME

Throughout this book, and especially in Chapter 6, *The Emancipation Equation*, I have suggested that one of the signs of true freedom is the acceptance of responsibility. Alongside this I have also argued that our tendency to think in terms of dehumanising abstractions like 'the system' allows us to more readily essentialise and demonise out groups and, in turn, to blame them for many, if not all the ills we believe beset us.

As I write, the *vogue du jour* in mainstream cultural and political discourse in the West is solidifying around the narratives of what we currently call identity politics, populism and entitlement. Not only does this point to an uptick in broadly ideological thinking and the generalisations and name-calling this tends to imply, but this often virulent trio underscore and attempt to legitimise our commonplace habit of blame shifting. In tandem with the mono-causal fallacy this has also created fertile ground for the righteous self-flagellations of middle class guilt; that overfed alt-pose of the shame-faced oppressor who just wishes they were cool enough to be poor, disenfranchised and statistically likely to die twenty years sooner. (If only they could put down their iThing for a second and go without food for a month they might just crack it.)

Some of the more popular examples of *you're totally to blame* and *oh my awful shame* include:

160

- It's the migrants' fault we all lost our jobs.
- The patriarchy is entirely to blame for me failing to get whatever I want – and wants to rape me.
- The feminazis are entirely to blame for me being hopelessly single – and want to castrate me.
- As an affluent, straight white guy I feel the need to apologise for every injustice that ever befell anyone (except guys like me).
- You are poor and voiceless because leftist elites hate you.
- White men are systematically defrauding, denying and disenfranchising you.
- Us white guys get blamed for everything – and dammit I've had enough and I'm gonna say so.
- The Islamisation of the West will mean the end of fun – and the genital mutilation of your daughters.
- PC queers want to destroy the family unit and steal everything you've worked for – and force your children to cross dress.

Of course there are countless variations on this theme, and not all are as hysterical as the examples listed – and indeed, as noted elsewhere, injustice, prejudice and nastiness continue to exist. However, my intention here is not to tick or cross particular iterations of blame/shame but to draw attention to the underlying similarities that these kinds of narratives share.

Looking at them from the outside, we see that these constructions all rely on the use of labels and, more particularly, on the delineations of groups within society and the subsequent ascribing to those groups of characteristics, intentions and actions.

Whilst there are those who would seek to entirely demonise our proclivity for labelling, it should be noted that our pattern loving brains have been driving us to slice and dice our perceptions and categorise our experiences since well before any military industrial complex ever got started. It certainly didn't take a gang of rich banking magnates to invent in group/out group distinctions. Neither did it require a sexist paradigm for us to recognise gendered behaviour differences, nor mainstream media for us to understand that some children are born with physical and learning difficulties that greatly increase the burden of care.

Therefore, to suggest that our tendency to name stuff (to label, categorise and delineate), is inherently oppressive is yet another ideological over-read. That said, like any tool, our sifting and sorting capacities can be used unwisely and unfairly. In the case of the current fashion for 'identity' it is being used as a crude mechanism of us/them division; and we see this trend reflected in the sound-bite polemic of modern politics and in the 'blame & shame' populism of social media feeds.

Here again we encounter the usual suspects:

- Dehumanisation and demonisation.
- Mono-causation and narrative reduction.
- Historical amnesia and the refusal to consider evolution and animal fact.

The febrile tone of so-called gender politics in the twenty-first century West offers us perhaps the most clarion example of this one dimensional blame/shame dynamic. Both sides routinely fling insults – rapist objectifier, guilt tripping castrator – and both steadfastly refuse to acknowledge that both men and women hold sexist views and act in sexist ways. Neither seems ready to allow that the other is also affected by restrictive gender stereotypes. Meanwhile, feminists (including its many male proponents) tout the all-round superiority and sanctity of women as a plainly evident truth and, as if in response, those in the men's rights camp (including women) wail about PC censorship, male disposability and systematic emasculation.

In my view, both are engaged in an unedifying yelling match, where the prism of gender is used to propagate all manner of narrative excess. Even though both camps shine a light on the unfortunate and often cruel results of standard gender and sexual memes, the current tone of gender identity politics borders on extremist idiocy. (This despite the fact that, since the days of Mary Wollstonecraft (1759-97), Western feminism has contributed significantly, even heroically, to the recognition and subsequent unleashing of the capacities and contributions of fully *half the population* to the cultural and economic life of our societies.)

But of course the attraction of this crudest of dichotomies is really that all the participants get to shift blame, externalise responsibility, play the victim card and remain in a childlike state nearing slavery, where vile overwhelming forces mitigate against them leading the life they want and force them into servitude and/or shame. (And, if one is being *really* honest, much of the gender diatribe is doubtless informed by conclusions drawn from painful personal encounters, broken hearts and bruised egos.)

Let's be straight: in the well fed, comfortably housed, historically liberal-minded West intellectually sustainable excuses for blame and shame have worn very thin indeed. This is not to say that there aren't good fights left to fight and excellent fighters left to do the fighting, but rather that the easy linear attractions of infantile storybook encapsulation more often win the day and that, with the microphone of social media ever ready, the loudest cultural noises are the braying sounds of locked horns and the tabloid tantrums of grown up children.

When we really drill into the sandpit dramas around identity and entitlement what we witness is a kind of ring-fencing. Territory being demarcated. Teams being picked. This harks back to the notion of the clan, which distinguishes itself from others, defines its membership and stakes out its ground; better to defend itself against external threats. Perhaps if we weren't living in such mammoth denial we would be able to clearly recognise these basic social animal traits in our abstracted and supposedly civilised behaviour – and maybe, just maybe, find mechanisms of belonging that weren't so rooted in fear and exclusion, nor indeed be so slavishly reliant on use of the command and control narratives.

But then again, maybe that's just me being fanciful. ☺

APPENDIX 2.
MY PHI

or

Turning the blowtorch on myself

Like most of us, I was an ambitious young thing.
At one point, like a lot of teenage lefties, I think
I genuinely harboured notions of 'saving the world'.

Having used fictional examples in Chapters 2 and 7 to tease out the implications of my informal happiness equation – the Potential Happiness Index – I thought it only fair to consider a real life example; namely, myself.

Quite apart from any possible conceit on my part, (I mean, why would you be even vaguely interested?), I trust that this exercise will underscore once again the deeper purpose of the PHI. Embedded in the construction of the equation is the idea that there are multi-variate inputs that affect our choice making and either contribute to or detract from our overall sense of wellbeing and self-authorship. In other words, we all wrestle with conflicting impulses and deal with variable socio-economic and environmental/circumstantial conditions against a backdrop of fluctuating health and a steadily diminishing fund of time. However, what the PHI process does is to quantify, to make more conscious, the connection between how much value we place on each of the various inputs – or how important we think each one is to us – and how this then affects our potential for happiness. Basically, the PHI is a kind of happiness math; an algorithm to help underpin your ongoing existential investment strategy.

Earlier in the book I created cut-out caricatures called CEO, Bourgeois Buddhist and Jan to flesh out the idea. These were deliberately clichéd confections, even a tad extreme, but now that we've come to examine a complex, inconsistent and decidedly real person the stakes are higher. So, just as it was for my fictional figurines, the challenge here is to be fearlessly honest. There is no point me lying to myself, nor indeed to you. In fact, here is where I get to put into practise, and print, a bunch of those 15 Things I talked about in Chapter 10.

Okay, so before I dive into autobiographical detail, here's a quick reminder of what the PHI looks like.

$$PH = \frac{\frac{\left(\frac{C}{T}\right) + A + Eq}{\left(\frac{V}{R}\right) + \left(\frac{O}{E}\right)} + W}{T}$$

PH = Potential Happiness

C = Capacity (overall health)

T = Time remaining (estimated in years)

A = Sense of Achievement

Eq = Equanimity (sense of calm & balance)

V = Validation (need for)

R = Relationships (importance of)

O = Obligations (importance of)

E = Ethics (importance of)

W = Wherewithal (finance, networks, conditions)

In the interests of transparency I should add that although I have declared in these pages and elsewhere that I am the happiest I have ever been, I did not directly utilise the PHI to arrive at this pleasing state. If anything, it was the other way round.

It is perhaps also fair to confess that I have come off a fairly low base, happiness wise. Without getting into the drama, I have done the depression thing, visited the well of despair and, yes, not just contemplated but actively planned suicide. (A bridge, a fast flowing river, a foreign city.) I mention this not merely to sound alarms or trumpet exhibitionist honesty but to suggest that my currently good frame of mind exists within the context of an often fraught past and, of course, an uncertain future. You may make of this confession what you will.

THE PSEUDO-MATHEMATICAL LIBERATION OF A FREELANCE BOHEMIAN

As I am fond of saying, I have lately come to both create and practise an 'economics of doing whatever I want'. It's a big claim, so let's see if the numbers really stack up.

Here goes … ☺

C: Capacity – expressed as a percentage.

Back in Chapter 2 I suggested that although I'm tempted to opt for 80%, reality and other aches – not to mention palpably failing eyesight – mean that the truer figure for purely physical capacity is most likely sub-70%.

However, given that I get around in a fairly unhindered way and can still do almost all of what I enjoy without unbearable agony, *and* that I have no burning ambition to scale mountains, take up jet skiing or represent Australia at badminton, my slowly diminishing bodily capacity is offset by a very healthy mindset and a vastly improved and far less self-immolating attitude.

Thus, on reflection, and balancing out body/mind/heart/etc, I'm going to score C at **75%**.

T: Time remaining – numbered in years.

Here we come to the most valuable asset I have at my disposal, my existential currency. Time is literally what my life is made of. To live, to be aware, to have a self, is to exist in time.

As I type I am in my early 50s and I …

- Am in relatively good health – no chronic ailments, not overweight, okay blood pressure, etc.
- Come from two generally long-lived lineages – maternal and paternal.
- Don't often engage in high risk consumption activities like tobacco smoking, guzzling fizzy drinks and eating fat drenched, super-sized servings of Mc-junk.
- Moderate my recreational drug use – including both alcohol and processed sugars.

- Enjoy the benefits of daily walks, sporadic dancing and brain exercising activities – like writing this book, learning guitar and keeping up with digital technology.

- Am in the best mental health I have ever been.

- Live in a locale (St Kilda in Melbourne) where people don't shoot and stab one another that much.

- Live in a country (Australia) with a decent and reasonably functioning universal health and welfare system – and, y'know, sane gun laws and stuff.

Given all this, I'm figuring that I'll make it to at least 90 before I'm either dead or incapacitated to the point where suicide once again becomes a live option (so to speak). However, for ease of calculation I'm going to nominate a big T number of **37.5**.

A: Sense of Achievement – on a scale of 0-10.

Like most of us, I was an ambitious young thing. At one point, like a lot of teenage lefties, I think I genuinely harboured notions of 'saving the world'. (I know, ridiculous, right?) Then, as a self-declared 'creative' I worked, with varying levels of energy and commitment, towards the goals of publication, recognition and credibility. Later, I strived to get film and TV projects off the ground. Along the way I veered from the jilted arrogance of the unheralded genius to the lacerating self-loathing of the out and out failure, traversing almost every possible point between – including real jobs, paying clients, a marriage, a mortgage and a dismal attempt at telemarketing.

However, after a particularly traumatic and ego-shattering episode in my mid-thirties, I consciously began the process of de-coupling myself from the lure of external validation (success, fame, cash, chicks, etc). As with any addiction the recovery program was a steady, trial and error journey; starting with bold and repeated assertions and evolving thereafter into deeply embedded daily practise. However, it was only when the declarative, determined force of intellect was matched by the sheer power and stunning clarity of emotionally 'getting it' that ambition (and its partner in crime: crushing self-doubt) finally and honestly withered.

Shortly thereafter it occurred to me that I was living more or less exactly the life I had so long dreamed of; that of a freelance bohemian, not shackled to a 9-5 grind or a mountainous mortgage, not begging at the altar of approval or status, and free to pursue projects of my own invention for ends of my own choosing. Okay, so I'm not loaded, don't own a bunch of stuff and have pretty well zero profile in my chosen fields – yet even if this represents *empirical, real world failure* my attitude to it is such that it feels like satisfaction, liberty, wealth and happiness. Indeed, even if forced to confess that all I've done here is cobble together sweet sounding justifications for a fundamental lack of talent and perseverance, I still *feel* great. I'm still writing this book because I love both the process of its creation and what it says to me about the kind of guy I am and the mode of living I enjoy. Because, if I have one ambition left*, it is to do whatever I want and be in alignment with the authentic inner self/voice I discussed in Chapter 10. The rest, quite frankly, borders on utter irrelevance. In light of all this, my sense of achievement number is a very satisfied **9**.

(***** Okay sure, I would also like to get better at guitar.)

Eq: Equanimity – on a scale of 0-10.

As you might imagine, for someone with little or no remnant ambition the equanimity thing is easier than it would be for someone still earnestly and feverishly striving; if only because a whole raft of frustrations (and the should narratives underpinning them) have been removed. However, to suggest that equanimity is simply a lack of desire, or just settling, would be to sell it short.

Equanimity is less about blithely not caring and more about understanding when and how much to care; or when to struggle and when to let go, when to gracefully accept defeat and how to be gracious in victory. I like to think of it as a kind of balanced perspective. Like taking a long position in the existential marketplace. A calm, considered outlook tinged with a healthy dose of humility and acceptance. Sorta like that famous Rudyard Kipling poem everyone loves to quote:

> *If you can dream - and not make dreams your master;*
> *If you can think - and not make thoughts your aim;*
> *If you can meet with Triumph and Disaster*
> *And treat those two impostors just the same …*
> – from: *If* (1895)

Most of us like to believe that we're pretty good at the Kipling-meets-Buddha mature understanding routine. I am no different in this regard. Of course, this makes scoring the Eq a little tricky. For instance, how much of my apparent equanimity is delusional – a self-serving bias that impels me to think rather well of myself? I mean, maybe I'm really just an out of control drama queen in an *haute boho* pose. Perhaps this book is a torrent of menopausal crackpottery totally divorced from anything even remotely resembling reality. Shit, this paragraph could even be a desperate cry for attention disguised as self-effacing 'meta' cleverness. *Arggghhhhhh!!!!!* And so it goes.

So, instead of winding myself up in knots of pantomime analysis, or resorting to the odium of comparing myself to others, I have elected to score the Eq on the evidence of observable change. In other words, am I getting better at this? Looking back at the me of ten years ago I'd say yes indeed. As for the Paul of the year 2000, 1991 or 1985, well … does *OMG fuck yeah* cover it?

I suspect that this is true for most of us over forty. Equanimity is a corollary of the years. Thus, with all due modesty and a pinch of salt, I'm allowing myself an Eq score of **7.5**.

V: Validation – on a scale of 0-10.

As I suggested in Chapter 2, I will publically confess to a V number of **2.5**.

Partly, this decision is driven by the same self-serving bias radar I mentioned above, but also because I, like you, am a social mammal. For all my declarations in this book I do not – and do not wish to – live in a lonely void. Therefore, I will not pretend to be entirely above the satisfactions that flow from the friendship and approval of others. In addition, I will admit to utilising the moderating presence and opinion of significant others as an orienting reference point and useful anchor. They are my human fail safe device, a GPS for navigating the shared terrain of our lives.

And y'know, should an attractive woman ever smile becomingly at me ever again, I'm sure it will make my day.

R: Relationships – on a scale of 0-10.

Evolved sociability and romantic disposition notwithstanding, relationships are less important to me now than ever before. Indeed, as I have progressively culled and curtailed friendships – both personal and professional – I have become happier. These days, spending time by myself is just about the most relaxing and rewarding investment available. I go to shows and movies alone, I eat out solo and, in fact, this very evening I'm off to see one of my favourite Aussie bands without the tiresome bother of a plus one.*
(* The Jezabels at the St Kilda Festival. A twilight set, no less.)

That said, (and using the risk/reward prism), it is worth remembering that fully-fledged misanthropy is a pathway to bitterness and distorting isolation. After all, it's a sweetly balanced 'sustainable solitude' I am aiming at here, not the life of a crazy curmudgeon squatting in a stinky bachelor cave festering in over-thought scorn. Furthermore, there is mounting evidence that, as we age, social contact is a critical factor in maintaining both mental and physical health. And then there's the sheer delight to be found in the company of our furry and feathery friends. All of which leads me to plump for a fence sitting R number of 5.

O: Obligations – on a scale of 0-10.

Okay, I'll be frank, I do *not* feel obliged. I do however willingly and consciously take on certain obligations – I meet my deadlines as a journo, observe share house niceties and strategically attend selected meetings with gruesome marketing sorts – but I do all this knowing I could just as easily choose not to. Here again, cost/benefit comes into play. In addition, I gladly factor in a broadly based obligation to humanity and society and therefore refrain from gang violence, sexual predation, sociopathic manipulation, and from the wanton waste of resources and the careless pollution of the biosphere so prevalent in the First World. Boiled down to pithy encapsulation this roughly equates to an obligation mantra that sounds like: a) do unto others, b) there but for grace of God go I, and c) leave it as good as you found it, if not better.

None of which, when examined honestly, is actually obligation. It's *all* choice. Because, in the historically privileged twenty-first century West, obligation is primarily for slaves. For all the sinner/victims out there. For the system blaming, custom upholding abdicators of responsibility. For the ideologues and demagogues who want to reduce the world to simplistic certainties and, by extension, control you.

Still, in the spirit of equanimity and with one eye on the next section, let's agree to a modest O number of **1.5**.

E: Ethics – on a scale of 0-10.

In Chapter 9 – *Ethical Investment In A Meaningless Void* – I outlined my reasons for observing moral principles. The question here though is how much value do I ascribe to ethical consideration when making life choices? Do my ethics censor me, stop me having fun or being true to myself, or do they prudently guide me, reminding me that I can actively contribute to the social contract and to the creation of a culture of trust? Does morality let me live at peace with myself, those I care about and the world at large?

As a self-declared Existentialist-cum-Nihilist I am principally *a*moral. I understand that all the value judgements we call morals are anthropogenic, socially sanctioned mechanisms for moderating individual behaviour within the context of herd survival. What's more, commonplace morality has been co-opted by the parental/external authority complex to bolster power cliques and underscore cultural orthodoxies, often with cruel and idiotic results. Through this prism I have come to view my own ethics as being driven largely by self-preservation, risk metrics, notions of character, empathy and, dare I say, aesthetics.

So yes, there are still lines in the sand – not many, but still very evident – and these ethical markers do influence my behaviour. Indeed, they are still actively informing behaviour change. On this evidence, I will score E at **3.5**.

W: Wherewithal.

Whilst previous sections focused more on the internal, this one goes external. By wherewithal I mean practical capacity to act in the world to achieve objectives. This takes into account the socio-economic, ecological and cultural conditions that affect us all and, significantly, our attitude to such things.

As part of the PHI I have formulated wherewithal as $W = En(F+N)$ – which means:

- En: Prevailing environmental conditions – good or bad? – expressed as a percentage.
- F: Finances – healthy or not so? – on a scale of 0-10.
- N: Networks – useful insiders or decorative outsiders? – on a scale of 0-10.

Turning first to the EN part of the equation, I am at once deeply concerned – unsustainable economic practise, spectacularly stupid mainstream cultural noise, the stubborn persistence and near ubiquity of slave and should narratives – and yet somewhat philosophical. I am effectively inoculated against the maladies of dystopian/apocalyptic paranoid despair, or the adoption of blind faith in tech fix panaceas and messianic redemptions, by a predominating view that if humanity is too arrogant or myopic to work out how to live together in synergy with its biosphere, then the process of evolution will prevail to arrange either a mass cull or extinction. Humanity and the civilisation we have created have no divine or other right to prevail. Sure, I'd prefer it if my fellow humans could work their shit out but, put it this way, I and no one else will miss us if we fuck it up. So, for En I'm opting for a moderately upbeat **60%**.

As for finances, on one hand they appear dire. Most people I know earn and have access to substantially more money than I do. However, since my last regular job got axed when the 2008 Global Financial Crisis obliterated the economy of the tropical tourist town I was operating from, I have learned the liberating skill of living on very little. (Or going without, as my gran used to say.) The whittling down of my apparent needs and an attendant reduction in my wants, coupled with astute budgeting, has helped to ease me off the spending hook; meaning that a small and sporadic freelancer income now stretches quite far. In this regard, I consider myself relatively wealthy. I mean, I live what many would consider to be a fabulously carefree life in a groovy inner city, beachside burb. Therefore, raw numbers notwithstanding, I'm giving the F a score of **5.5**.

Networks, on the other hand, are not so great. I possess no old school tie, am not pals with the powerful, have no famous friends and, as I mostly operate solo, have no workplace web of handy contacts. Being honest, my network score is **2** at best. This then gives me a final PHI scorecard of:

	SCORE	
Capacity	75%	
Time remaining	37.5 years	
Achievement	9	
Equanimity	7.5	
Validation	2.5	
Relationships	5	
Obligations	1.5	
Ethics	3.5	
Wherewithal *	4.5	* as a result of $W = En(F+N)$
Environment	60%	
Finances	5.5	
Networks	2	

Calculated to three decimal places on a very clever phone, my PHI number is 0.65104, which then translates as a **65.104%** chance of sustainable happiness going forward.

LIVING BEAUTIFULLY WITH 65

It may well be argued that 65% is not that flash. You may indeed point to my relatively subdued wherewithal number and suggest that my love of the low-fi lifestyle wires me into a sub-optimal existence. Maybe if I worked a bit harder and did the networking thing better more doors would open for me and … so on and so forth. I could even try being friendlier, putting more emphasis on relationships or, heaven forfend, get some more solid ethics happening. Fuck it, I could take up gym membership or give up cheese.

And my answer would be *yeah of course I could do more of this, less of that, and give these things a good tweak.* In fact, further fine tuning is inevitable – because what I have here (with the PHI) is not the immutable result of a mid-life exam paper but a useful quantification that prompts me to ponder again the value of my belief portfolio and how the choices I make about how to live and what to emphasise might affect my chances of genuine happiness.

Therefore, as I write today (on a lovely blue sky Tuesday morning) I am neither euphoric about nor crushed by 65%. In fact, given that life is riven with uncertainties and unknowables and that circumstances can change abruptly, my PHI result strikes me as a definite win. With my risk/reward goggles on, I am satisfied that my current existential market position is structured to deliver a long term dividend flow and to make my journey to the grave more pleasant than unpleasant, and to leave me feeling more liberated than incarcerated.

To me, 65% is the beginning, a reference point. Maybe I'll look back on this one day and think how miserable I seemed then, or how complacent, how stupid, how absurd. Or indeed, how fortunate. I cannot *know* this. I only know that time will deliver its measure of shocks and surprises, that there will be wins, losses and draws, and that I will age and die. All that truly matters to me right now is how beautiful the unfolding process will be – and how I can best contribute to that living beauty.

APPENDIX 3.
MY BEAUTIFULLY POINTLESS EXISTENCE

or

How I learned to revel in futility & embrace the void

To put it another way, I did not *fight* for freedom,
I surrendered for it. And because I did not
seek a cure I made myself well again.

In this Appendix I dig into the autobiographical detail. Though this is at least partly due to latent exhibitionism, my intention here is to place all my previous contentions in their genuine context; namely, a human life. To that end, I present the story of 'surrender' and 'the ecstasy of nothingness' and the narratives that drove me to become both fully accountable and happily free.

- Beginning with an act of surrender
- Revealing the ecstasy of nothingness
- The archaeology of surrender & ecstasy

   +

- The beautification of everything

In Chapter 10 – *The Authenticity Channel* – I hinted that, aside from there being rational observation based reasons and practical techniques to help us focus upon and disentangle our true voice from the incessant noise of socio-cultural background radiation, there also exists a quieter, perhaps more 'mystical' means of identifying and remaining in clear contact with the authentic (self, soul, spirit, instinct, etc). Here too, I am referring to the process (and experience of) unearthing powerful change agents and sources of motivation in the metaphysical/spiritual space and, furthermore, suggesting that what I discovered there amounted to a revelatory and convincing piece of my personal liberation puzzle.

I stress that what I'm about to discuss is merely my idiosyncratic take on things and that no copycat profundity or epiphany is either compulsory or required. *The Pointless Revolution* mandates no spiritual practise and sets no minimum enlightenment standards. What's more, I am not purporting this to be the revealed truth, nor indeed any kind of divine or cosmic wisdom – let alone the meaning of life. In its simplest form what follows is a metaphysical map reference, a deeply enigmatic and beautiful note to self. As such, it underscores the more intellectual arguments I have made in this book and reminds me (via the experience of ecstasy and awe) why I have chosen the way of meaningless being.

BEGINNING WITH AN ACT OF SURRENDER

In order not to drag you through the minutiae of my 'spiritual journey' I will jump cut straight to a pivotal moment when, at 42, I made the conscious decision to break with a lifelong tradition. Without wishing to sound heroic, it was probably the gutsiest thing I ever did, the single biggest risk I ever took. I knew what the potential costs were but I had a very deep sense, bordering on knowing, that the old techniques would not suffice.

Basically, I was in yet another shit-hole of despair – episode whatever in a repetitive saga of heartbreak and so on. The same old girl trouble, only this time in hyperdrive. The order of magnitude, in pain and 'crazy-thinking' terms, was a step change up from anything I had dealt with previously. I was out of control, in freefall, and I had just enough remaining smarts to know it. I won't lie, it was alarming. At times it was like, *whoa, is* this *who you are?* Yet, a decade on, it is now clear that both the form and the overwhelming intensity of the situation was the culmination of a long-running self-drama that involved all manner of delusional narratives and habitual behaviour. In a way, the lady in question was an innocent bystander.*

(* For a fuller back story and even more grizzly personal details, see below in the section marked: The Archaeology of Surrender & Ecstasy.)

One night, shortly after things had 'turned to shit', a concerned friend was doing his best to placate and persuade me with all the usual self-help style remedies – this platitude, that suggestion, blah blah – but even though I could see the ordinary sense in what he was saying I knew that this time they wouldn't work. After all, I had been employing a wide range of self-awareness/self-talk methods to medicate and minimise my various angsts and effectively 'therapise' myself since I was a hormonal teen and, to be fair, these modalities had proven largely successful in bandaging my collected wounds and keeping the show on the road. But I knew that there was no talking this one neatly away. The usual pills of polite, middle class pop-psych were not even going to touch the sides this time.

My reply that night, as near as I recall it, went something like this: *I dunno, I think I have to walk through the fire this time, not round it, and if I get burnt, I get burnt.* As soon as I said it out loud it was as though the idea coalesced, took understandable form. Over the next few weeks it firmed into an action plan of sorts.

Surrender.

Whilst I understand that 'surrender' sounds a tad dramatic and militant, I chose it precisely because of this. It was far less beige than safe sounding bourgeois terminology like 'letting go'. Its very power said something about the process involved that 'letting go' just didn't, and still doesn't capture. Furthermore, 'surrender' felt like it demanded more of me, pushed me further. At the end of the day, all I can say is that it was the right choice for me. Aesthetically, spiritually and practically.

In a way I was being fatalistic, throwing myself into a churning river. However, with hindsight I can see now that what I was doing was learning to trust the needle on my inner compass, my deepest instinct. Rather than the reduction of words or theories, or the hubristic and righteous assertion of so-called wisdom, I was going to let the fire burn what it may. After the flames, I would deal with whatever was left – unless of course I got burnt to cinders in the meantime.

Looking back at those first fiery weeks from the safety of ten years, I understand why my initial act of surrender was so pivotal. When, as everyone tends to, my helpful friend eventually said, 'Hey, y'know you'll be okay, don't you?' I knew with astounding clarity that he was wrong. Surrendering the complacent conceit of 'being alright in the end' opened the door to what I now regard as a truly transformative experience.

I was effectively allowing, rather than controlling. Dropping the legislated, complacently assumed outcome meant that all possibilities were on the table. By agreeing to risk everything, not only my high functioning public edifice but my sanity more broadly and, ultimately, even my life, I was giving permission to the deconstructing scalpel of despair to cut away my protective, obscuring layers and reveal the form beneath. What transpired was a massive shedding of skin. Eventually I was naked before myself. A frail ape with pretty language and big ideas. A walking smorgasbord of habit, assumption and longing. An intricately patterned incidence of atomised, self-recognising consciousness. No longer the inviolable young thing of photographs and glory-tinted nostalgia.

This first act of surrender then rippled out into:

- Abandoning the notion of self-importance.
- Challenging and disempowering the habituated rituals of vanity.
- Confronting and overcoming the often unconscious addiction to status and objects.
- Disavowing righteous conceit – abandoning salvation crusades and enlightenment journeys.
- Busting long cherished self-mythologies – and other ideological addictions.
- Confronting patterns of denial – fearlessly poking around in the dark.
- Disempowering punitive self-judgement narratives – ejecting the right/wrong, pass/fail dichotomies of the parental/external.

Then, in the day-to-day, surrender soon began to ring in the behavioural changes:

- Simplifying my lifestyle – not taking on so much, not wanting so much spectacle and excitement.
- Getting rid of stuff – letting objects go, buying far less, etc.
- Dealing sooner and more decisively with tyrants and abusers – becoming clearer about who I would allow to get close and in which relationships I would invest my time.
- Recognising my own patterns earlier, thereby creating opportunities for conscious choice.
- Divorcing the drama – less distracted by the various spectacles of self – gaining clearer perspective on setbacks, traumas, etc.
- Letting go far more easily – not holding on so much – going with the flow more – moving on, etc.
- Living much more in the present – and with the increased gratitude and moments of joy it can entail.

At this juncture it is worth clarifying two key aspects of surrender. Firstly, I was not surrendering *to* something, per se – except perhaps to the notion of my own ephemeral and infinitesimal existence. This loss of self-importance, this almost cosmic perspective on self, felt like being in the presence of a blind, and therefore egalitarian, immensity. Secondly, all of the above flowed from the darkness; not from battling it, nor from pathologising and opiating it, but from walking willingly into it. Indeed it is my current belief that by plunging completely and without a safety net into the dense wave of despair – by accepting that it was neither bad nor noble, but that it was simply a momentum, an event, and that I could just as easily choose to let it drown me – I was delivered to a fount of ecstasy. For in the black, all sources of light are obvious.

To put it another way, I did not *fight* for freedom, I surrendered for it. And because I did not seek a cure I made myself well again. By dropping all pre-ordained objectives, value judgements and lazy assumptions, and setting aside the various projects of the ego, I arrived here: at the door of happiness, humility, gratitude, clarity and equanimity. With a 65.1% PHI score. Without mandated alpha objectives to fret about, destiny to realise or externally authored moral checklists to tick off – just an amount of time to invest in doing whatever I want. The sheer minimalist simplicity of it brings a smile to my face.

If surrender proved to be the big trigger for my recent and ongoing liberation it also kickstarted a programme of psycho-emotional weight loss. Most of that heavy old shit I was heaving around – objects, habits, sacred cows, etc – I just let drop. These days, there is so much less clutter in my head and in my house, and so much less baggage to carry in my heart.

But it wasn't all about jettisoning the junk – because I found, or rather unambiguously identified, the authenticity channel. This was the voice that urged surrender. That said *forget all that fucking noise*. That lifted my eyes from the melodrama of a highly poeticised sorrow (call it an artistic mid-life crisis) with a bold but gentle promise:

- Surrender … and you shall be free.

Though it may be impossible to entirely capture the essence of surrender in words, suffice to it say that it is (somehow) so much more than meek capitulation to a higher power, or simply giving up. It is a kind of *active* acceptance. Active, not in the sense of blocking and denying, but in being absolutely alive to the unfolding process of inevitable change. Of being fearlessly fluid. Radically light. Of accepting with grace that all outcomes are ephemeral, save for the final one. To surrender is to be supple like the reed which survives the storm, as opposed to rigid like the oak which snaps in the high wind.

To be frank, once you've started down this path, the dictats and imperatives of the parental/external get put into perspective. It soon becomes difficult to take their bucket lists and sinner/victim mantras seriously. Eventually, the 'should police' lose their coercive power because as soon as we detach from caring about their objectives we begin to regard them as either unimportant, dysfunctional or fear based control mechanisms. The plethora of 24/7 socio-cultural channels seem much less significant and, in fact, become so much background babble. From there it's easy to just tune them out.

REVEALING THE ECSTASY OF NOTHINGNESS

However, beyond surrender, I have lately stumbled upon a form of mystical, metaphysical experience that offers to open up yet another channel – to ecstasy and awe and, thereafter, to an oceanic compassion. True, these feeling states belong entirely to me; they spring from and form part of an ongoing and particular anthropocentric interpretation. Yet simply feeling them has proved nothing short of profound. I am not alluding to a Godhead moment or to the revelation of the deep secret or ultimate key to everything, but rather to an experience of transcendence which underscores, in the most extraordinarily simple and beautiful terms, all my intellectual reasons to be free. In a way, this newly discovered experience is the bonus ecstasy dividend of my long term surrender investment.

Although the first inklings occurred way back in my teens, and hints got dropped across the decades, I was fifty when it eventually distilled into the big 'ringing of the bell' moment. And the trigger for and focus of this beautifully vibrating epiphany? Perhaps it is merely an idea, an abstract plaything or mathematical object, maybe even a Platonic form; or then again, it could be part of a fundamental existential paradox – like the impossible inevitable or timeless eternal. Either way, I like to think of it as The Nothing.

My introduction to this mystical 'Nothing thing' happened in the back of a mini bus.* I was working on a film project, being driven to a remote location, when the cast and crew drifted into one of those D&M, 'this is what I really believe' conversations. It was fairly predictable stuff – everything happens for a reason, my soul is on a glorious, ascendant journey, etc – but it was what happened next that took my breath away. Literally. I was wondering if the others would ask me to join in, although somehow I knew they wouldn't, and so I posed a question to myself, 'What will you say if they ask you?' A beat later I had my answer, which seemed to drop out of nowhere. 'I would say that I was an Ecstatic Nihilist.'

(* The fact that, a few days previously, I had played a part in saving a young man's life had obviously put me in the right frame of mind for such an epiphany. I'm sure you can imagine why.)

Upon uttering those words in my head I was suffused with an immediate, electric, breathless wave of what I can only describe as euphoria or awestruck ecstasy. (Writing about it now, my body tingles, hairs on end.) Abruptly, everything was still. Silent. And I was looking at the Void. As near to being outside myself as I had ever been. Closing in on the paradoxical axis of everything and nothing.

In what seemed like an incredibly long space between breaths I found myself focusing on the notion of absolute nothingness and a voice in my head said, 'From the unity of The Nothing you came and to it you shall return.' I recall being flooded by a mentholated tide, like a quiet monolithic immensity washing right through me – and it felt in that moment like an infinite form of love and compassion; and I knew at once that there was nothing to fear and that, as such, I was completely free.

A couple of years down the track, and having had many similar experiences of what I now call 'the ecstasy of nothingness', the plainest explanation I can come up with is that these episodes are like an asymptotic approach to an impossible vantage point – or space, or realm – one beyond that ordinarily available to iterated identity complexes like you and I. It is a perspective that no human, no individual living consciousness, can fully access. Indeed, if we must think of it in personalised terms (as seems to be our habit), any being or consciousness enjoying such a vaunted perspective would not even be an atomised self-identifying I, and as such would have no subjective position, no plans and no opinions and, what's more, would 'exist' outside time. They would, in fact, have no life or death as we normally conceive of them. In short, the nothing p.o.v. is the view from the outside of everything. The view from stillness.

Of course, boiling this down into the linear form of human language is bound to create problems. After all, how can we describe The Nothing? Or is the word 'nothing' really the right one? However, getting tied up in semantics and pedantry is beside the point because what all these words are pointing at is an experience, a knowing, a profound liberation. In Chapter 10 I used the phrase: *it is the deepest of deep backgrounds, the very canvas upon which the splatter of our existence is cast*; but we might also say things like:

- It is the silence that listens.
- The emptiness that contains.
- The stillness we move through.

Or, for those of who prefer it in more personalised deity terms:

- It is the divine absence.

Poetic paradoxes notwithstanding, the roll out of this mystical experience has manifested as the deepest peace, sweetest joy and most complete freedom I have ever known. In The Nothing all distinctions melt, all grandiose declaration is silenced and all judgement is suspended. When I contemplate The Nothing I am reminded again that none of what I think matters *actually matters*, and that all of humanity's Gods, karma committees, destiny narratives and meaning tropes are fictions. Denials. Thus, the ecstasy of nothingness is the complete dissolution of mortal dread, the 'as near as it gets' transcendence of self, and the subsequent and sheer relief that flows from the abandonment of meaning. It is the *Pointless Revolution* as a breathless, electric vibration.

After the euphoria of emptiness, well … each time I am free to begin again. Tabula rasa, terra nullius. Almost newborn.

This, combined with the practise of surrender, represents the core metaphysical underpinning and deepest motivation for the things I have discussed in this book. My investment in these seemingly mystical meanderings has delivered the most powerful and happiness-generating stream of returns I have ever known. For what it's worth, I can thoroughly recommend them.

THE ARCHAEOLOGY OF SURRENDER & ECSTASY

NB:

Quite clearly, there's a whole line of philosophical and spiritual inquiry in this surrender and nothingness business. In fact, another book. However, cute theorising aside, my embrace of the act of surrender and my being alive to the moment of ecstatic, back-of-bus 'revelation' were seeded in much less academic soil. They sprang from personal history and, of course, from the story of self I have been developing over the course of my conscious life. Indeed, to be absolutely brutal about it, most everything in this book has emerged from (and is a retro-fitted explanation of) deeply personal and often conflicting proclivities and desires – and they, in turn, are a response to the discreet circumstances of my life. For just as others seek happiness and/or solace via an edifice of essential meaning, or seek to anchor and orient themselves by endless reference to externally validated measures, I have engaged in my self-declared *Pointless Revolution* for similar reasons. Because I wanted to find a way to live and now, at last, I am happy with what I found.

So *how* did I get here?

From the hindsight of fifty-something it is easy to see the patterns that have played out (and still operate) in my life. The loops and iterations, the biases and addictions, my persistent desires and the repeated dramas they generate. For, like you, I am a creature of entrenched habit. Indeed, that tired old phrase, *the more things change the more they stay the same*, most definitely applies. Even the life-altering shifts in behaviour and awareness I have detailed in this appendix and elsewhere have flowed almost seamlessly out of old cycles. More than once during the process of writing this book I have caught myself midstream and thought, *hey, isn't all this just* that *old thing?*

As for the patterns themselves, they clearly evolved and became embedded as the result of a myriad of circumstantial factors; some external and beyond my control and others more endogenous. Aside from the usuals – genetics, gender and physicality, upbringing, socio-economic conditions, cultural context, early socialisation experiences, dramatic and disruptive events, etc – the foundations of my ongoing story of self are to be found in everything from pop songs and paganism to leftist/humanist ethics and acts of homophobic violence (of which I was intended victim)*.

(* Observant readers will have noted references to an ex-wife and other lovers of the womanly variety; yet, hetero though I am, I was – as a teen with a funny haircut and an obvious love of 1980s pop androgyny – the local 'fag'.)

Clearly, in the service of brevity, I am not going to bore you here with endless, self-obsessed detail (like that last bracket). So, rather than an exhaustive life story, I will focus instead on the seventeen key repeated narratives that informed the very notion of 'the character called Paul', some of which still drive important life choices and underwrite core beliefs. These narratives have lately coalesced into a story of beautifully pointless liberty; yet although they now form the basis of an existential wealth fund that generates significant happiness dividends on an almost daily basis, for decades they were part of my investment in misery, impotent rage, intellectualised posing, righteous vanity, and a virulent strain of guilt, self-loathing and punishment. (Perhaps you will recognise some of these in your own story of self.)

- The narrative of otherness & exceptionalism – I am not like other people, so therefore …
- The narrative of defiance & rebellion – I do not have to obey or be like other people, and so …
- The angst of unfairness – I have been dealt lower scoring cards than most and am at a structural disadvantage through no fault of my own – constant struggle against the odds – eyesight-related frustrations.
- The 'getting away it' strategy – if I'm smart and careful they'll never find out – bluffing and subterfuge – lies and denial – storytelling and 'work arounds', etc.

- **The drama of self-loathing** – not only am I let down and constrained by my 'faulty' body and relative unattractiveness but am obviously an immoral person – a skilled liar, a well-spoken fraud, a snob, arrogant, lazy, accomplice to the oppression of women, ignorant Westerner, passive-aggressive manipulator, and so it goes.

- **The drama of noble suffering** – my pain makes me better, smarter, worthier – suffering is beautiful and uplifting – suffering is artistic – happiness is shallow.

- **The narratives of compassion & justice** – we should not be judged and condemned for things we can't help – we are all flawed and, therefore, worthy of kindness, understanding and forgiveness.

- **The 'teacher/saviour' pose** – with my superior wisdom and compassion I will lead you into the light – which in turn will help me feel useful and loved – rescuer/hero fantasy – messianic conceit.

- **The 'artist/authority' pose** – with my superior intellect and creative brilliance I will inspire you to save yourself – which in turn will win me admirers (perhaps even lovers) and, importantly, help me to like myself and trust my judgement more – benevolent, far-sighted genius fantasy.

- **The narratives of realism & acceptance** – I understand that there are forces I cannot control – certain limits have been externally imposed – some fights aren't worth fighting – reality does not always accord with the dream; the fact of which can be a source of both relief and humility (and even a convenient excuse).

- **The narratives of improvisation & transformation** – give me a bunch of ideas, even half-cooked, and I can make them work – we can turn our hurdles into assets, our lack into plenty – we can work both within and without the rules – a limitation, viewed creatively, can become a freedom – pain can be transformed into beauty.

- **The narratives of humility & gratitude** – the world is brutal and uncaring and, thus, I am fortunate to have what I have – I am not special, just lucky – I do not regret – I cherish the simple things – this is not mine by right, I enjoy it by the grace of happenstance – everything can be taken away in a trice.

- **The animal fact** – we are but one of many species on this planet – civilised humanity is a veneer – so much of what we do, say and pursue is a form of lie and denial – our deluded arrogance is destroying us collectively and saddening and enslaving us individually.

- **The and/also view** – there is no single encompassing answer/way/reason – I myself contain contradictions – apparent opposites can also be viewed as the same thing – the multi-perspective view – pluralism, relativism, etc.

- **The unknowable future view** – all decisions/plans are a form of risk – lets cross that bridge when we get there – despite the best laid plans – stay fluid, etc.

- **The 'perspective' prism** – how small and insignificant we are in the grand scheme – how short our lives are – this is just an episode – this too shall pass – these are but trinkets, etc.

+

- **The tinted lenses of beauty & romance** – there is a better world – there is a more beautiful way – there are people out there who will allow me to love them and/or love me in return – and even if there aren't we shall persist anyway; because to do otherwise is to give in to fear, cruelty and ugliness (and we will not knowingly contribute more of this shit to the world).

Suffice it to say, I could fill up several pages with further examples but the list above gives you a fair indication of the multiple and interwoven narratives that laid the groundwork for both the surrender episode and the nothingness moment and, beyond that, much of the focus and distillation of thinking that has led to this book. What you may also have noticed is how common many of them are and also how contradictory. Indeed, some sit in almost polar opposition. Again, many of you will be familiar with the everyday fact of wildly conflicting desires and ideas. My guess is that, if we're honest, we can all confess to being consistently inconsistent.

Thus, despite my almost life-long delusion of exceptionality I suspect that much of the above will resonate (including the exceptional bit). I say this to underline once again that the happiness and lightness I have found is not the result of super-human effort or talent. I have conquered no peaks, visited no ashrams, been anointed by no deities. Money and formal education have played little or no part – and in fact may even have been a hindrance at times – and glittering socially visible success and other trophy moments have been notable only by their absence. In addition, my current contentment is not a reward for moral uprightness or clean living discipline. Like most of you, I am neither a paragon of virtue nor an especially egregious sinner. Therefore, despite still being deeply attached to my treasured otherness mantras, I am equally convinced of my utter ordinariness.

At this juncture, some of you will doubtless be sensing a humility connection; namely, that being humble made the act of surrender and the dropping of self-importance easier. This is true. However, for me at least, being humble is also about being real. It's just plain practical, if only because it dilutes the disappointments and reduces the amount of time and energy involved in trying to hold onto stuff (especially vainglorious fantasies and entitlement claims). Indeed, I was in my early twenties when I realised that nothing was so sacred that I couldn't just let it go. Later in life I came to apply this to long-standing beliefs, ambitions and assumptions. Not to mention so-called friends. Indeed, even before the surrender drama began, I was versed in the art of de-cluttering – having already off-loaded most of what I owned, abandoned a safe job and a beautiful seaside residence, and walked away from the harmful juvenile fantasy of justice, fairness and general human goodness.

NB:

This is not to suggest that people are generally 'bad' but rather that humans, myself included, are principally self-serving creatures, unconsciously driven by evolutionary/animal/survival factors. Furthermore, we are limited, flawed, opportunistic and largely unreliable. Rather than pathologising this I simply accept the plentiful evidence of it as a little more than a map-read. In this way moral judgement is rendered irrelevant; so too the persecution and entitlement narratives that so often go with it. Prior to letting my youthful 'people are all good' fantasy drop I was constantly smacking my head against a brick wall of unmet expectation, outright betrayal and attempted predation. In a way I was victimising myself, repeatedly salting the cuts because I was needy, because I was looking for others to convince me I was an alright guy. And so they treated me as badly as I let them. These days though, my guiding mantra is more like: people are people, deal with it.

But of course, the impetus for surrender was not just a measure of judicious humility or the targeted disposal of excess baggage, nor even a thicker skin. For it to be anything more than a dry, intellectual exercise I needed to be addicted to the siren songs of unrequited love, poetic agony and mutual exceptionalism. Hence, for the surrender girl and I, our shared 'beautiful suffering' narratives and a *contra mundum* (against the world) attitude were slammed together like fissile material in a reactor of sex, recognition and almost deliberate self-destruction. Right from the start there was a fatalistic wantonness about it all. I knew she was dangerous, that I would almost certainly pay a high price, but still I went ahead. 'My eyes are open,' I told myself. In reality, they were open just enough to put me on notice.

That the subsequent affair involved a former student twenty years my junior, that she was clearly a survivor of various abuses, and that her emotional antennae seemed to twitch just like mine … all these things just added to the fire. Made it wild. Yet, whatever else has been obscured in memory or mythology, she and I shared a deep connection – a connection that somehow went right to the core of me. In fact, right through me. Fanciful though it may sound, I often think that it was the children in us that met. I will not speak for her but what I saw in her was, in a very real way, a vision of myself. A perverse and dramatised vision certainly but a reflection nonetheless.

But she wouldn't let me save her – so there was nothing for it but to save myself. That I elected to do it without painkillers, bandages or any kind of safety net was, in a way, typical of our doomed rebel drama. *Death if need be, but never be like them.*

At any rate, that was my read; and yes, I *am* prepared to admit that it was completely delusional and that my recollection of it is skewed and self-serving.

Nonetheless, setting aside the swoon of hormones and the couple bonding tendencies of the human animal, the experience of her advent and her 'inevitable' leaving was the most intense, far-reaching and dangerous drama of my life thus far. She was, to some extent, the apogee of several of the narrative strands listed above; even if it was never her intention. Insofar as she was an agent of change, it was more like a dark serendipity; it just happened to be her who triggered the castle's collapse. Fortunately, I knew this even at the time.

This understanding was critical. *It's not her, it's me.* Then, following on from that, another key realisation: *I can choose to put off looking at this or I can deal with it now.* Typing these words today it abruptly occurs to me that surrender began when I finally took full responsibility. When I *owned* the despair and, simultaneously, allowed it its full expression without either glorifying it or beating myself up over it.

If she was the mirror, I was the wild-eyed stranger staring back. From the safety of ten years, I can speculate that perhaps, subconsciously, I was attracted to her because I knew that only the way to disarm my increasingly harmful addictions was to ramp up the agony. To drive myself to the edge. To make denial and dithering untenable. To force a choice.

Set fire to everything. Work with whatever doesn't burn.

I realise how reckless and extreme that sounds – how dramatic – but it worked. Surrender prompted a full-scale reappraisal and, as the heartbreak trauma slowly waned, a thorough and unblinking yes/no/maybe process of psycho-emotional closet clearing kicked in. It certainly wasn't plain sailing but I am reaping the rewards right now.

Yet, even as I gained new clarity and unwound the coils of narrative habit, my suicidal ideation grew both more persistent (daily) and less emotive. In the weeks leading up to the nothingness epiphany detailed in the previous section, I hatched a cold, rational, cost/benefit plan for one final act of self-obliteration; and although flight bookings and filming itineraries effectively thwarted that specific plan I knew that I had found a model for a clean suicide that would either look like misadventure or leave ample scope for plausible doubt.

In effect, as I was sitting in the back of that bus in the moments before nothingness, listening quietly to the D&M burble of my companions, I had already arrived at an existential crossroad. Put simply, after all the post-surrender analysis, I was consciously weighing the options thus: is it worth staying alive for another forty years of this?

I knew I could carry on out of sheer habit, or indeed to prevent the suffering of my parents and others – although, to be honest, that 'suicide is selfish' thing never really cut it with me.* Therefore, if I *was* going to choose life, it may as well be a happy one, as opposed to one mired in the values, beliefs and meaning tropes that had underscored such persistent misery and punishing self-denial. Given that, I may as well structure my life with deliberate focus to increase the probability of said happiness. If that meant abandoning cherished ideals, walking away from work projects, cutting certain people out of my life and giving up the pursuit of women, then so be it. Similarly, if it meant taking a punt on passion over profit and professional development, or if it pushed me to prefer the risk of colour over the safety of a beige consensus, then all I would require was both the spine to say yes and the honesty to own up. In the end, when I *did* choose life, I chose liberty – and in this way, surrender ultimately delivered on its promise of freedom.

(* I have no 'issue' with suicide whatsoever. For me, if there *are* such things as rights, the primary right is the right to choose *not* to live. If we're blackmailed into staying alive, we're slaves; and if we're only alive because we're terrified of the alternative, our lives are effectively underpinned by fear.)

In this light, the 'ecstasy of nothingness' moment is less of a blinding flash and more of a confirmation. After all, I had long since rejected any notion of personalised Gods and had moved significantly beyond the commonplace fear of death. On top of that, the surrender process had cured me of ideological fixations and proved to me, in stark and powerfully emotional terns, that the parental/external authority complex relied on little more than bullying and bribery.

The nothingness event was the big dramatic pay-off. A confirmation in the form of absence. An absence of command and control. Of reward and punishment. Of pre-ordained objective and mandated outcome. In the Nothing there are no chains; and the never ending/never beginning circle of zero is indivisible. Is a unity. Is a oneness.

Climbing out of the clouds, for a moment we can interpret the Nothing mantra as a refinement of existing narratives and a philosophical justification of certain key psycho-emotional drivers. For even the most rarefied and pristine abstractions, the most Tao like and Nihilistic ideas are etched into the ordinary grit of self and most often serve its purposes. Or at least, they do in my case.

As an illustration, the last ten years of surrender and nothingness have coalesced into the following five headline narratives:

- Only in liberty can I make optimal life choices and act with complete honesty and commitment in pursuit of my objectives – anything less is a combination of de-motivating compromise, dishonest sell-out and self-punishment.

- My sense of liberty (and authorship) is best generated and sustained in the absence of Essentialist meaning tropes and predetermined life outcomes – if life is an exam or things are 'meant to be' then I am reduced to a child-like state of either parent-pleasing supplication or mechanistic box ticking.

- The meaningless life is the only one I would stay alive for – because its value does not derive from its relation to external sources of validation or its degree of compliance with socially or cosmically mandated criteria – its value is entirely self-generated and exists *in the present* – thus, for me, 'meaning' (or whatever you want to call it) is rooted in process, not outcome.

- How I feel (and how I feel about myself) is paramount – happiness over wisdom, contentment over apparent success, freedom over finance, integrity over vanity, compassion over cruelty – I need to like myself much more than I require anyone else's approval.

    +

- In the space vacated by traditional alpha meanings and 'whole of life' objectives … beauty.

What you will notice, even in this distillation, is the echo of older narratives, most notably defiance, otherness, perspective and transformation. To be an Ecstatic Nihilist who embraces surrender and is awestruck by The Nothing is, therefore, not as outlandish as it might otherwise seem.

Even beauty, which for me is an absolutely central value, makes much more straightforward sense when considered against a backdrop of being the puny, squinty-eyed, blind kid that the pretty girls passed over and the cool boys kicked away. From a very young age, without fully knowing what I was doing, I began to refine the art of transforming a sub-optimal world into something more tolerable. Initially, I looked for ways to fit more seamlessly into a world I couldn't quite gel with, before changing tack at thirteen and doing the outsider thing, effectively turning my pre-pubescent hurt and incomprehension into a triumphant badge of adolescent honour. By the time I had endured my first agonising and failed attempt to act as liberator (for the 'fallen angel' German girl in my Year Eleven maths class) I had already come to understand that the most unrelenting pain could be regarded as the most exquisite beauty. That despair was a gateway drug to a kind of euphoria.

All very teenage and purple, but it underlines something salient about my private *Pointless Revolution*. It was, at once, an act of emotional and intellectual subversion *and* conversion. It was both an overthrow and a reshaping of old forms, a transfiguration that described an arc from self to self. I *feel* completely different – astoundingly and wonderfully so – but I know I'm the same. It's just that now everything is much more beautiful.

THE BEAUTIFICATION OF EVERYTHING

So, what do I mean by beauty? Obviously I am not referring to the mere airbrushed prettiness of models or the Instagram loveliness of sunsets, nor indeed to any culturally sanctioned norms around what *is* and *isn't* beautiful. Instead, I am speaking of the 'deeper experience' we all have of beauty – those moving, nigh transcendent moments of appreciation, or of profound connection and gratitude, and sometimes even of seeming perfection. This is the stuff of songs and inspiration, of poetry and wonder. For me, the experience of beauty is, and has often been, what we might call profound. More than that, transformative. A refuge. A channel of salvation.

Given the scope and tone of this book, with its accent on practical, existential liberation, it has not been entirely appropriate to dwell too long on the topic of beauty. However, since we're at the end, I shall indulge, if only to share with you one of the more enigmatic triggers and sustaining sources of the life-changing happiness that inspired me to start writing this book.

If you read the previous sections, where I spoke of surrender and the ecstasy of nothingness, you may well have guessed that beauty is the third of a somewhat mystical triumvirate. In the absence of classic alpha objectives or standard life meaning stories, beauty is the nearest I have to a philosophical raison d'etre or, more poetically, a guiding light or higher ideal. Although I sometimes characterise beauty as my muse, I would hesitate to suggest that it sits in the 'god seat'. That said, when I'm really on fire, I am in the habit of personalising 'her' as Beauty and I will confess to being utterly in awe of and in love with her. (No, really.) Indeed, it is to her that I sometimes surrender and, in her arms, experience a sublime ego-less state of presence and flow. I have even used the word 'grace' to try and describe it. At cooler temperatures, like now, I fudge it a little, preferring to suggest that beauty is a kind of language, a way of seeing, of reconfiguring.

Should you be sensing a little vagueness on my part, well yeah, I am conspicuously reticent to reduce beauty to a rigidity. For I do not behold beauty as a thing (even when I pretend she's Beauty) or even as a definite quality that can be measured. Beauty remains outside the scope of words, beyond the language of maths, even though both words and mathematics can be experienced as profoundly beautiful. Beauty can never be entirely 'defined' or nailed down – and this, of course, if you'll pardon the pun, is an essential part of its beauty. Like The Nothing, it has the magical, paradoxical quality of being both knowable and unknowable. If beauty is the form of the good, it is also formless.

However, before we drift off into pseudo-guru levitation land, let's draw it back to this: in terms of human life beauty is both a value measure and, more importantly, an *experience*. The world itself is neither beautiful nor ugly. Electromagnetic frequencies and vibrating molecules do not, in and of themselves, possess aesthetic qualities or goodness. Data is just data. However, when that data flows through the prism of our consciousness, it is sometimes interpreted as being either beautiful, plain, ugly, etc. Beauty is anthropogenic, an entirely subjective read, and like kindness and honesty it is a quality we value; some of us more highly than others.

Whereas others will fixate on notions of objective beauty – referring to golden ratios and/or insisting that Beethoven, Renaissance art and trees are beautiful by definition because they supposedly accord to certain standards, or are just really popular – I prefer to think of beauty as a mode of *experiencing*. In other words, beauty is not external to us; beauty is a response we sometimes have. Not simply a value judgement but a *capacity*, a mode of perceiving. Perhaps because evolution has endowed us with a penchant for patterns and a complex sociability, as a species we have developed an ability to regard certain experiences as being more or less beautiful. These experiences typically include everything from the purely aesthetic (visual, sonic, textural) to the kinaesthetic and tactile (touch, taste, motion), as well as psycho-emotional states (love, contentment, melancholy) and the purely intellectual (ideas, solutions,

185

equations). Then of course there are the more spiritual beauty experiences, like ego transcendence, absolute presence, awe and ecstasy. And so the list goes on. Add or subtract what you may.

My interest here isn't the mere delineation of what can and can't be experienced as beautiful or the precise defining of its scope, but in the evolved capacity itself. I mean, why do we find things beautiful at all? Does beauty have telos? Even if we say that our talent for beauty is either an adaptation that somehow aids our survival or is an evolutionary anomaly, the fact that we are able to regard *anything* as beautiful is, in my view – apart from being really fucking beautiful – one of the most amazing, mysterious and value adding aspects of human existence. I mean, what an extraordinary thing for an ape to be able to do; not merely to survive, function well enough and pass on its genes, but to experience certain phenomena as being beautiful. Perhaps, ultimately, to regard its own simian existence as a thing of beauty.

To use myself as 'example ape', one of the things that helped me survive years of despair intact and to emerge from decades of emotional habit happier than ever was my ability to *transform it into beauty*. To find the beauty in stuff and, in particular, the dark and painful stuff. Although such psychological prestidigitation was once as an adolescent art pose, over the years the development and refinement of the beauty lens has enabled me to find beauty in a whole lot more than the sugar pretty or the obviously spectacular. By the time I was editing print publications in my early thirties a photographer friend of mine had already noted my tendency, as he put it, to elevate the mundane. Or, to beautify the ordinary. From there, by increments, I learnt to behold the beauty of less. Of emptiness. Of silence. Of the light itself. And of the fall of shadow.

Whilst this may sound like purist, minimalist, elitist art wank – and sure, sometimes we can lurch – it also underscores a much more dangerous but ultimately pragmatic response to dysfunctional behaviour patterns and increasingly suicidal despair.

As previously discussed, for many years I loved my own sorrow and had seemingly locked myself into an addiction relationship with misery, (depressed was so much a part of *who* I was, my drama of self), but eventually it was the sheer bittersweet glory of it, its puissant and brutal immensity, so like an ocean …

Hence, surrender – and in the thrall of that particular wave, where to yield to drowning is to be lifted up, I knew beyond any vestige of doubting that ecstasy and despair were the same. That it is from the heart of darkness that the beautiful light shines. And it is only our ego and pettiness and fear which prevents us from knowing its obliterating, liberating magnificence.

I realise how extreme this will sound to most of you, which is kinda why I saved it till now, but I cannot tell you how profoundly confirming and altering, how seismic, how absolutely beautiful it was. In fact, typing out that last paragraph? Tears of euphoria.

This is what I really mean by beauty as a transformative experience, as a manner of beholding. In many ways, beauty is *felt*. Known. But also it is an *act* of feeling and knowing. The experience of beauty creates the world anew and can reconfigure our role within it. This is why, for me at least, it is as close as it gets to what many call the divine.

Put it this way: beauty isn't so much *in* the eye of beholder; rather it *is* the beholding eye. Beauty *is* the prism.

So why beauty, Paul? Why not blither on about truth or justice, or even love?

Of course, if I'm being honest, I have to confess that my beauty thing is, as much as anything, a habit that began when I was very young, so young that I cannot clearly recall a first moment of thinking *ooh this is for me*. It was only as a self-conscious high school kid, inspired by idols (David Sylvian, Lord Byron, Charles and Sebastian from *Brideshead*) that I consciously and deliberately latched onto the notion of beauty as some kind of higher ideal. Yet it was another twenty years or so before I gained a proper understanding and full acceptance of how I had been unconsciously using it to both heal *and* further inflict myself. From that point, it was a relatively short stumble to the well of ecstasy and despair, and to the liberation it subsequently fuelled.

Again, sparing you the indulgent autobiographic detail, once my reverence for the 'ideals of beauty' had finally moved beyond the pitfalls of hauteur and drug-like dependency, I was truly able to say to myself *beauty is everywhere, you only have to notice it.*

On the face of it, this may seem like limp New Age cliché but, I swear, I am not about to start bathing everything in patchouli oil and declaring that all is wonderful and beautiful. Neither am I for one moment suggesting that any of us should whitewash our experiences and the wider world in a froth of legislated positivity bubbles – because, for me, beauty transcends all commonly understood positive/negative dichotomies. So, when I say that beauty is everywhere I am not saying that everything is good (as in cheerful, positive, not painful, etc). Nor indeed am I suggesting that it *necessarily* operates as a saviour and/or life affirmer. Beauty is not a cure in the narrower sense of well/unwell, for it does not pathologise.

Here then is the nub of it for me, and why beauty qualifies in my universe as the principal ideal, as one of the topline reasons for staying alive; or indeed as a form of what we might even call meaning. Once we get to the point where our sense of beauty encompasses more than simple good looks or the catechism of shiny happy affirmation, and when we *really, deeply* get the beholder/beholding thing, it can become a transcendent and transformative mode of experiencing. A window that lets us see beyond the blunt socially mandated dualities of everyday narrative. One that renders nigh irrelevant the crudities of pass/fail and the exigencies of status and attainment. That sees clear through the diaphanous conceits of apparent wisdom and the hubristic postures of enlightenment crusading. That melts the standard linear meaning tropes of 'about' and 'for', effectively de-coupling process from pre-ordained outcome and shifting the focal point of purpose from functionalities and future goals to a heightened present. Without wishing to sound *toooo* lofty, beauty is a form of gratitude, a kind of thanks for the Here & Now.

However, although we may regard beauty as a prism of value, and that in our beholding role we are therefore automatically making a judgement, this act of discernment does not (although it can) rest upon moral or ideological notions of goodness or rightness. Nor indeed does it stem from perceived utility or health and wellness function. Nor even from our narrowly aesthetic penchants for stuff like symmetry, violins or aquamarine. Because – tautologous and paradoxical as it sounds – the purpose of beauty for me is, if anything, simply to *be beautiful*. Just as the putative 'point' of existence is to get on and do some existing.

So now, after much to and fro and a lot of habituated posing and self-mythologising arrogance, I have come to understand myself as the prism shaper, as the one who does the *transforming into beauty* through the twin acts of deciding and allowing. More than that, by abandoning the reductionist safety of either/or and withholding judgements rooted in fear and control, the act of beautifying the world has granted me access to a range of experiences that offer a glimpse of something beyond the silo of self. Beyond grasping and achievement and the pedantries of so-called truth. Beyond me wanting to convince you.

In that spirit, and in conclusion, let me finish thus:

> *In her presence I am fully present, absolutely alive, and in that presence … absent. For to be with her is to be her, to blur the line between the I and the other and to melt, just for a moment, into the ocean of everything and nothing.*

Now *that* is beautiful.

ABOUT THE AUTHOR

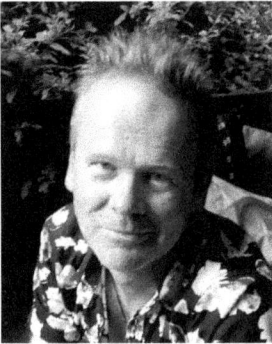

Paul Ransom was born in Brighton, England in 1965 and moved to Adelaide, Australia in 1972. After growing up in outer suburbia he married and tried to be a proper adult. He taught prisoners in a maximum security gaol, worked as a rock journo, film critic and magazine editor, did short stints as a nightclub DJ and band manager, and then almost passed for normal whilst working as a lecturer in the media/arts sector. After the marriage ended he absconded to the tropics, where he went without nice shoes and edited local publications for three years, before relocating to Melbourne to successfully complete a mid-life crisis and become an award-winning independent filmmaker. He has published literally hundreds of articles for various publications, made four very arty rock videos, released two unheralded (and frankly awful) novels, written reams of copy for countless clients and created a blog consisting entirely of love letters. He currently lives in a low rise 1930s apartment building and refers to himself on LinkedIn as a freelance bohemian.

ACKNOWLEDGEMENTS

As this is a non-academic book, there is no exhaustive reference list. However, I have clearly been inspired and influenced by writers, thinkers and close associates in the formulation of my ideas and their representation in text.

On the purely philosophical front I would like to thank my lifelong friends Dr Arthur Witherall and Guy Phillips. For economic insights my gratitude goes to my 'finance gurus' Tim Langdon and Robert Edge. For psycho-emotional smarts, eternal thanks to my ex-wife Ebony, our former therapists Dr Sandy Litt and Eugene McMahon, my 'psychologically savvy' friends Matt Cahill, Josephine Cox, David Willey and Alida Tomaszewski, and my insightful and compassionate mother Rose.

However, aside from personal nods, it's only fair that I tip my hat to the following:

Writers: Stephen Pinker, Thomas Piketty, Susan Cain, Felix Martin, Niall Ferguson, Mervyn King, Anatole Kaletsky, David Graeber, Richard Wrangham, Bertrand Russell and E.F. Schumacher.

Also: Lisa Cairns, David Eagleman, Marina Abramovic, the BBC World Service, Bloomberg News, PBS Space Time, Wikipedia (of course), and dead folks like Alan Watts, Terence McKenna, Friedrich Nietzsche, Maria Montessori and Lao-Tzu.

And lastly, for inadvertently prompting me to write this book, my fellow armchair philosopher and wannabe proletarian polymath, John James Ransom, aka – my dad.

Paul Ransom
Melbourne, Australia
Spring 2019

Your pointlessly revolutionary, low fat listicle

It was always the author's intention to keep this volume slender but, since wafer thin
is the new obese and the listicle is the social media equivalent of long form journalism,
here's *The Pointless Revolution* boiled down to a few 'feed friendly' lifestyle tips.
(I mean, why bother reading an entire book when you can ingest it all in fifteen seconds?)

———

Embrace your mortality with deep gratitude
Transform death from the source of ultimate terror into a licence to truly *live*, as opposed to merely staying alive

Revel in your infinitesimal and ultimately inconsequential role in the overall scheme of things
Live like no one's watching – because life is not a test and the universe is neither a judge nor a hero drama

Embrace the futility and emptiness of all striving and, consequently, disempower all success and status imperatives and the pass/fail judgements that go with them
Liberate yourself from the pressure of 'must' and license yourself to pursue genuinely rewarding, self-authored objectives

Resist the lure of Essentialist meaning tropes and the linear, reductionist simplicities of destiny narratives, higher purposes and grand cosmic/moral dramas
Throw off the shackles of standard, command and control, pass/fail meaning stories and author your own meaning-proxies
in the here and now without the sword of judgement and punishment hanging over your head

Locate the source of joy and reward in process and present feeling state, as opposed to future dated outcomes, trophies, cool cred and other forms of external approval
Delete the bucket list, throw out the must-haves, free yourself from dependence on either/or outcomes
and, of course, disobey the lifestyle police

Embrace uncertainty, admit ambiguity and always allow space for nuance, rule bending and incompleteness
Accept with equanimity that you do not, and will not know everything and that 'perfection' is not possible

Use a topical risk/reward prism rather than a rigid ideological filter when assessing life choices
Accept with equanimity that all choices involve potential costs and benefits;
and don't allow seeming imperfection to stymie decision, hold back progress or supress experiment

+

Regard your remaining time (what's left of your life) as your most valuable asset and, using the 'time as money' metaphor, invest only in what you believe will deliver 'value for money'
Become an existential economist

Or, if you want it even simpler:

Surrender
Be grateful
Be humble
Be accountable
Embrace the liberty of pointless being
(And remember, time spent will not be refunded)

ALSO FROM EVERYTIME PRESS

https://everytimepress.com/everytime-press-catalogue/

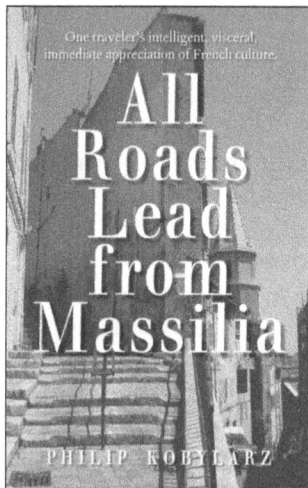

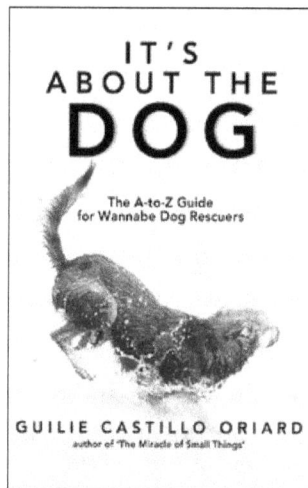

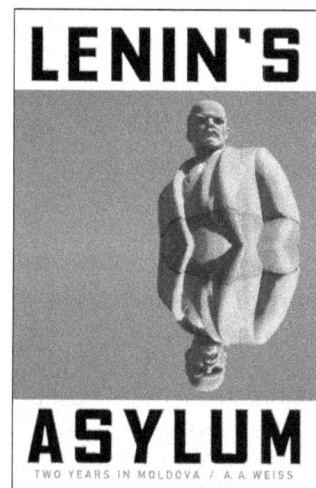

- All Roads Lead from Massilia by Philip Kobylarz
  978-1-925536-27-0 (paperback) 978-1-925536-28-7 (eBook)
- It's About the Dog by Guilie Castillo Oriard
  978-1-925536-19-5 (paperback) 978-1-925536-20-1 (eBook)
- Lenin's Asylum by A. A. Weiss
  978-1-925536-50-8 (paperback) 978-1-925536-51-5 (eBook)

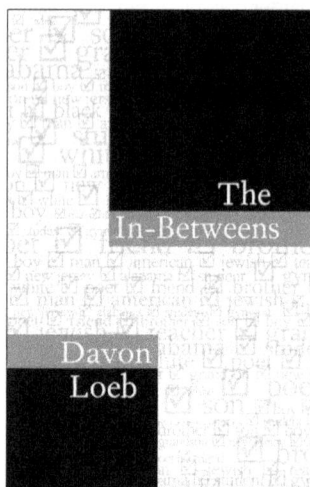

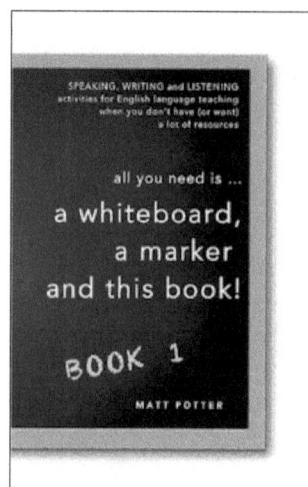

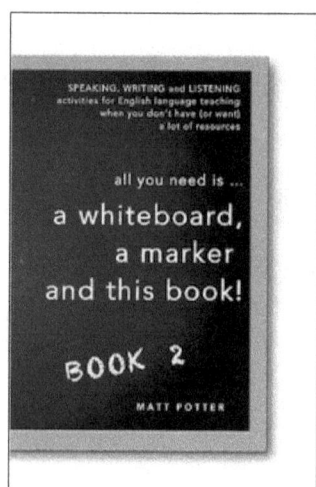

- The In-Betweens by Davon Loeb
  978-1-925536-56-0 (paperback) 978-1-925536-57-7 (eBook)
- all you need is … a whiteboard, a marker and this book!
  by Matt Potter   978-1-925101-82-9 (Book 1) 978-1-925101-96-6 (Book 2)